THE LASER'S
EDGE

THE LASER'S EDGE

Revealing a new, safer and more effective arthritis treatment with no side effects

Dr. Jeremy Alosa, D.C.

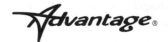

Published by Advantage, Charleston, South Carolina.
Member of Advantage Media Group.

ADVANTAGE is a registered trademark and the Advantage colophon is a trademark of Advantage Media Group, Inc.

Printed in the United States of America.

ISBN: 978-159932-423-4
LCCN: 2013943373

Cover photography by Justin MacKenzie.

This publication is designed to provide accurate and authoritative information in regard to the subject matter covered. It is sold with the understanding that the publisher is not engaged in rendering legal, accounting, or other professional services. If legal advice or other expert assistance is required, the services of a competent professional person should be sought.

Advantage Media Group is proud to be a part of the Tree Neutral® program. Tree Neutral offsets the number of trees consumed in the production and printing of this book by taking proactive steps such as planting trees in direct proportion to the number of trees used to print books. To learn more about Tree Neutral, please visit www.treeneutral.com. To learn more about Advantage's commitment to being a responsible steward of the environment, please visit www.advantagefamily.com/green

Advantage Media Group is a publisher of business, self-improvement, and professional development books and online learning. We help entrepreneurs, business leaders, and professionals share their Stories, Passion, and Knowledge to help others Learn & Grow. Do you have a manuscript or book idea that you would like us to consider for publishing? Please visit advantagefamily.com or call 1.866.775.1696.

Contents

IMPORTANT NOTE TO READERS

This book is not meant to diagnose, cure or prevent any disease. The evidence presented in this book is for informational purposes only. Many patients have been able to achieve long term pain relief from the treatment presented in this book but that in no way guarantees results of any kind for anyone. I have been given written consent to use each individual patient testimonial contained in this book.

Introduction

I first experienced severe pain when I hurt my back in college training for the coming football season. I had been sprinting and at the beginning of one sprint, I came out of my stationery position—and that was it: my back just locked up. I couldn't move. Somehow I managed to get myself back to my room and into bed where I stayed for two days. Physicians examined me and gave me pain medication that did nothing to help my condition. Every time I tried to move, a sharp pain would shoot down my back. I was in agony, thinking I would never be able to get on a football field again. I was ready to do anything, try anything, to ease the pain.

That's when my mother asked if I would see a chiropractor. I didn't know anything about what chiropractors did, but I said, "Let's do it." I remember I could barely get into the car or sit upright. When we got there, the chiropractor did a few tests. Then he adjusted my lower back. I was shocked; I felt instant relief! I was still sore, but within two days I was good as new and back on the playing field. I was elated when just days before I had been lying on my back, feeling hopeless.

The experience affected me profoundly: I realized how much of a life-changing difference someone can make helping others with their pain. I wanted to be able to make such a difference, so as soon as I graduated from college, I entered chiropractic school. After four years of study I earned my degree and eventually started my own practice. Over the years, as my practice grew, I noticed more and more patients coming to me for arthritis treatment. They were essentially in the same situation I had been in as an injured college football player: these patients had terrible pain or numbness and had come to a chiropractor as their last resort. They had already been to doctors who had subjected them to painful cortisone shots or surgeries that had provided only temporary pain relief. Now they were at a point where the doctors were essentially telling them they had to live with the pain because there was nothing they could do.

When I realized that people with arthritis had limited treatment options, I began to research an alternative for them. That's when I discovered one of the most effective treatments available today: laser therapy. Of course everyone knows about lasers; they've been around for a long time. But in recent years a particular laser, the class-4 laser (15 watt), has been found to be quite effective in the treatment of pain and numbness in arthritis patients. I began working with it in 2009 and was amazed at the results my patients experienced.

However, most people still don't know about this treatment or how or why it works. My goal in writing this book is to help you understand laser therapy so you can decide if it may be a possible course of treatment for your arthritic symptoms. My hope is to simply get the word out so more people can know what their full range of treatment options are. You will be pleased to discover that arthritis does not have to be the life sentence of pain that it used to be. There is definitely hope now, even for severe cases of arthritis. I have worked with such patients in my office and the laser therapy has gotten them better. People who have been physically disabled for 20 to 30 years can now walk without the assistance of a cane or walker. These patients discover, once their pain is gone, a new lease on life is created.

You will also find in this book a very candid discussion of how the health-care system works or doesn't work in the United States.

Many patients come to me as a last resort, but not because a doctor has sent them. In many cases the medications or surgeries the patients endured could have been avoided if they had tried laser therapy first. But that option isn't presented to them. You'll find here the reason our health-care system operates in this way so you can be a more proactive participant in the process. You can still go to the conventional medicine practitioner and listen to what he or she prescribes for you, but after reading this book, you will also know that you have other options such as the class-4 laser to treat your pain. With this information, I hope you will be able to make better decisions on how you want to proceed with your treatment plan. You'll see that being a more informed patient can make a very big difference in securing a favorable outcome for your condition.

Chapter 1

THE PAIN OF TODAY'S HEALTH-CARE CRISIS

A discussion of health care in America may seem like an odd place to begin a book about arthritis treatment, but you'll soon see it really is the most logical way to begin. In describing any kind of medical procedure these days, I think it is important for patients to understand the workings of the medical system. Most people have common misconceptions of the system and a troubling blind faith in doctors that, unfortunately, have become dangerous to a patient's health. Why? Because a lot of the decisions doctors make these days are not based on what is in the best interests of the patient. They are based more on what procedures doctors can do that will allow them to get paid the most.

Many patients, casting themselves in a very passive role, put their faith in their doctors and just take their word as law. They close their minds to other treatments, especially what they deem to be alternative health-care treatments such as laser therapy, because a doctor has not offered such treatment or even mentioned it to them. There is a clear reason why such treatments are not offered and it is important for patients to understand it.

HOW THE SYSTEM WORKS

When you experience a health issue, whether it is pain or nausea or general discomfort, the first thing you do—and most people who have health insurance do this—is visit your primary care physician. Most patients will go to the physician fist and wait to see what the MD tells them. From that basic starting point the patient can be funneled into a process involving a variety of medical procedures and treatments. But note: medical doctors are very reluctant to recommend an alternative health-care treatment such as laser therapy.

Typically, arthritic patients wake up one day with back pain. They go to their physician who may do a few tests. The physician will diagnose the arthritis and possibly prescribe a drug for the pain. He or she may even tell the patient to just live with the arthritis, that it is simply the result of wear and tear and part of the aging process. In short, you just have to deal with the pain. But let's say the drugs don't work, and for the most part, they never work because dugs can only provide temporary pain relief before ceasing to be effective. Then, the doctor may give you some cortisone injections or prescribe some physical therapy. If those options fail, the medical doctor has only one option left: surgery. A doctor may recommend surgery even when the patient is not an ideal surgical candidate. Why? MDs prefer to keep a patient in the medical paradigm or medical model. That medical model leads to invasive surgeries and dangerous prescriptive drugs that can actually cause a lot of other health problems down the road. Still, doctors are very reluctant to refer patients to alternative treatment services even though the options may be very safe and help patients to feel better.

Let me be clear about this: I don't want to give the impression that all medical doctors are bad people; far from it. They are simply functioning within a system and this is how the system works. For instance, medical doctors trained as internists look at symptoms, figure out what's going on, and decide whether or not a medicine can cure the problem. Surgeons are trained to think only in terms of "How can we cut it?" because that is what surgeons do: they cut. It is just the way the system is set up: doctors are trained in the one thing that they do, and this is the way they look at conditions, with a very narrow mind set, but not with any bad intentions. This is the way our very flawed medical system works.

WHY YOU MUST BE PROACTIVE

With a system so flawed, I would even say broken, patients are tasked with a bigger responsibility to think in their own best interests. If you, as a patient, are not proactive, you may be led away from a treatment that will work for you. I've seen this happen in my own practice too many times to count. When some patients under my care see their primary care physician and that doctor finds out the patient is undergoing laser therapy, the doctor tells the patient not to do it. The doctor even claims the treatment is not going to help, so the patient stops my treatment. When I call these doctors on the phone to discuss the treatment and the kind of laser therapy I use, I often find they know nothing about it. When I explain the different classes and types of laser, the doctors realize they were wrong to react so quickly. This is just an example of what I deal with in my office.

Imagine how many more times this happens to chiropractors and other alternative medicine doctors all over the country.

THE CURRENT HEALTH CRISIS

In the United States we spend about $2.6 trillion a year on health care, which puts us at number one in the world by a wide, wide margin. The country at number two, Japan, doesn't spend half of what we spend. But what do we get for all this spending? As it turns out, when you compare many of the U.S. health statistics to those of other industrialized countries around the world, you'll see that we perform very badly. We are spending a lot more money, but our health isn't better than anyone else's. In fact, our health in the United States is a lot worse than in most other countries. Cuba, for instance, has a better infant mortality rate than the U.S. rate. This sad state of affairs was reported in a landmark study by Barbara Starfield, entitled, "Is U.S. Health Really the Best in the World?" in *The Journal of the American Medical Association* (JAMA) in July 2000. If the health of the country kept getting better, that would be one thing, but to spend all this money and have the health of U.S. citizens only decline doesn't make much sense. It just proves that the system is broken.

Why do we spend so much for so little? Because health-care costs are spiraling out of control with no relief in sight. In this country we perform more invasive, expensive treatments, such as surgery as a matter of course, sometimes before even considering less expensive, less invasive options. In countries such as Japan, it is done the other way around. They consider the most expensive, most risky treatments last. But here in the United States, we usually cut first and consider everything else afterward. With just one visit, a family doctor may send a patient right to an orthopedic surgeon without even having the patient try physical therapy, chiropractic treatment, acupuncture, massage, or other treatments that are a lot less costly, invasive, and dangerous. When you go to a surgeon's office, the surgeon is usually going to recommend surgery.

If every patient with arthritis pain underwent laser therapy before going in for any kind of injections or surgeries, you would see costs in this one area alone come way down. Low-back fusion surgery on the spine can cost anywhere from $50,000 to $80,000. That's just for a surgery. It does not include all the outpatient care needed once surgery is done. Add on top of those costs the fact that 50 percent to 60 percent of the time the patient will require another surgery.

A MATTER OF LIFE AND DEATH

Here's what can happen when people do not understand how the medical process works. They go to the doctor's office with a painful knee. The next thing they know, they are talking to a surgeon and eventually undergoing a total knee replacement. Six months later, maybe the knee replacement didn't fit. Maybe it loosens. The patients go back and their doctor has to take that replacement out and put in a new one. The patients may still have knee pain because the replacement still doesn't work. Now, because the knee is still painful, the patient is compensating putting more pressure and stress on the surrounding joints, such as the other knee, the hip or the lower back. This extra load on the sorrounding joints will create arthritis in those areas! Now the patient has arthritis pain in multiple areas instead of just one.

Contrast this result with that of patients who know the process. Patients with knee pain go to their physician who recommends they see an orthopedic surgeon to discuss surgery. The patients may make that appointment, but because they understand what is going on, they may ask to try something less invasive, less risky, first, and then make their decision. They look into alternative treatments and decide to come to my office to try laser therapy. It works; the knee pain is better. They do not have the surgery, which means they will not have the side effects that would have come from the surgery.

In the end, such patients are much healthier for their good decision making, even more so when you consider this: it could be a matter of life and death. Many patients die from knee surgery, even arthroscopic knee surgery, a minimally invasive procedure. Infection is still a risk with any procedure and many patients contract and succumb to infection postsurgery. Every year some 80,000 deaths occur from hospital-caused infections. That may even be a low-ball number because the true numbers of infection probably do not get reported. But 80,000 per year is not a low number when you put it in this perspective: 50,000 people died in the Vietnam War and that was over the course of ten years! When you think of the risk, how willing are you to put 100 percent of your trust in your doctor to make the right choices for you and tell you the right thing to do?

MEDICINE AS A BUSINESS

The doctor doesn't have the patient's best interests in mind – but again, this isn't necessarily the doctor's fault. Medicine has become a business and a mammoth one at that. Most hospitals now are owned by corporations, and corporations' main goal, number one, above all else by far, is to make a profit for their shareholders. Patient safety is not a number-one priority, and probably not even a number-two priority. Patient safety gets pushed to the back burner if the corporation realizes, for instance, that it can implement a procedure that may be riskier than others but generates a lot more money. Sadly, it may be okay if a certain number of patients die because the amount of dollars the procedure is bringing in makes it worth the risk. That, unfortunately, is the state of health care and that is part of the crisis.

The Food and Drug Administration (FDA) feeds the profit machine as well. After denying drug companies the ability to market their products on television, the FDA in recent years gave in to company complaints. Now, commercials for pharmaceuticals clog the airwaves, helping to inflame health-care costs. Only the most expensive drugs are advertised on TV, but when patients see the plug, they immediately go to the doctor, demanding that drug. And there's usually no generic form, so patients come in asking for the most expensive drugs (which is exactly what the drug companies want). But this marketing tactic further escalates the health-care crisis without adding any benefit to the patient because there is always an older, generic form of the drug that is just as effective. The Vioxx debacle is a great example of this, and I will go over the details in the pages that follow.

So you have corporations **running** our hospitals and drug companies exercising a very, very strong say when it comes to medical care, what treatments are offered, and definitely what drugs are prescribed. These companies are obviously very powerful. They make billions and billions of dollars, and their reach extends further than you think: they can even influence the education of our physicians.

BIG BUSINESS EDUCATING DOCTORS

All doctors, once they earn their medical degree, must complete a certain number of continuing education credits just to maintain their license. But they don't necessarily have to enroll in school or university to earn those credits. In fact, in the medical field, the majority of continuing education seminars – where doctors can earn their credits – are all organized by drug companies. The drug companies pay for the seminar, they pay for the speakers, they pay for the materials, they pay for everything. So what does a doctor sitting in such a seminar learn? He or she is basically presented with a sales show by the drug companies; the presenters at the conference promote the drug company's drugs. The drug companies control the education the doctors receive about their products. The companies will also pay for doctors to be consultants for them, and often when doctors attend these seminars, it is the drug companies that pay the expenses, footing the bills for food and lodging, usually at very fancy five-star resorts.

At the seminars, these paid doctors will promote the drugs that the companies offer, presenting studies that are really just sales tools for the drug companies. The seminars are large-scale versions of what happens in doctors' offices every day of the week. Anyone who has ever been in a medical doctor's office may recall seeing drug company representatives, known as detail people. These detail reps meet with doctors and present research on their drugs. That's how a lot of doctors obtain their information on drugs. They are too busy to do their own research, so they have the drug company's sales reps come in and present theirs. Obviously, this is not an ideal situation. The research is biased and is presented only with the goal of making a sale. Unfortunately, the same thing happens when a doctor tries to do his own research and reads the leading medical journals. Many of the research articles in such journals are published or funded by the drug companies. When these companies pay for a research article, they will get the results they want and this is the reason, according to Dr. David Eddy, MD and his research published in the *British Medical*

Journal states that only 15 percent of research articles published in major journals are scientifically sound.

THE ROLE OF THE FOOD AND DRUG ADMINISTRATION (FDA)

One would think the FDA would play a very big role here in protecting the public against the marketing machine of the drug companies. That is what everyone perceives the FDA's role to be and that is, in fact, what it is supposed to be. Unfortunately, the reality is this is not the case. These days, the FDA is set up in such a way that a lot of the department's income is produced by the drug companies. How? Simply this: The drug companies have to pay to submit a drug for approval. The bulk of the FDA's income is derived from these fees. So the FDA organization is supposed to protect the public by policing the drug companies and regulating the drug companies, yet the drug companies are the ones who pay the FDA's employees' salaries.

Not only that, the same people who work at the FDA, once their stint with the FDA is done, usually go on to work for those same drug companies. They earn a very big salary in a big cushy job when they do so. It's like a revolving door. It's very hard for the FDA to regulate drug companies when they receive so much income from those same companies and when so many FDA employees plan to work for those drug companies when they're done with the FDA. As a result, the FDA does not effectively do its job of protecting the public or policing the drug companies. Instead, the FDA feeds the problem. Again, you can say the system is to blame. Just as the doctors in the medical system are forced to do things a certain way, so does the FDA operate to suit the system. This is why alarming situations occur with drugs such as Vioxx.

Several years ago Vioxx was touted as a blockbuster drug for the treatment of arthritis. It was supposed to be a great drug because before Vioxx, patients had to take nonsteroidal anti-inflammatory drugs, such as Aleve or ibuprofen. However, these drugs had a tendency to cause ulcers and bleeding in the lining of the stomach. Vioxx was supposed to be easier on the stomach, eliminating stress and damage to the stomach and the intestines. When that first drug first came out, if you went to your doctor's office with any kind of arthritis pain, you would have received Vioxx because it was the new, highly touted drug for arthritis pain.

Vioxx racked up millions of dollars in sales before it was discovered that the drug was causing heart attacks and strokes. Some 88,000 people died, but the FDA did not remove the drug from the market. The agency required the drug's producer, Merck, to change the labeling and advertising copy. The drug itself remained available. In the end, Merck, acting on its own and not at the behest of the FDA, pulled Vioxx off the market. This is a prime example of how FDA just doesn't do the things it should be doing to protect the public. Instead the department seems to act to protect the drug companies and their profits. Vioxx was just one example, but it is a very clear example of how the FDA fails the country as a whole. This is hard to believe but it is the truth and that is all that matters.

A lot of people took Vioxx and died from it because it was approved when it should not have been approved. When a drug goes through the FDA, its approval process only takes six to nine months. You can't properly test the safety of a drug in six to nine months. It takes years. In fact, it usually takes about seven years to know the full safety of a drug. The only way to thoroughly test any drug is through intense, long-term study. The drugs that are approved by the FDA are deemed safe and appropriate, but the reality is that the real testing only gets done when these drugs go out to the public. With Vioxx, this process failed miserably and 88,000 people died. Now contrast how the FDA behaves when the public seeks alternative care. The FDA can come down very hard on doctors working with cancer or arthritis patients, using treatments other than prescription drugs. In fact, the department has been known to go into establishments and confiscate all the doctors' materials, equipment, and case files. The doctors may go to jail, and the FDA can freeze all their assets. The department can do whatever it wants and has done so just because the doctors used nontraditional treatments—namely, no prescription drugs.

The FDA is obviously very powerful and going after alternative-medicine doctors is another way this power is often used to protect the profits of the drug companies. The FDA says these doctors are breaking the law. How? Because the FDA actually enacted a law that states that doctors can only cure or treat a disease with prescription drugs! The Food and Drug Administration says only a drug—nothing else—can cure, prevent, or diagnose a disease. Therefore, the Food and Drug Administration continues to call more and more and more ailments a "disease" and tries to eliminate natural remedies. No one can advocate a natural remedy if the ailment has been classified as a disease. So attention deficit disorder is now a disease. Therefore, only a drug can cure, prevent, or diagnose it. Osteoporosis is a disease. Acid reflux is now a disease. Obesity is now a disease. Any doctors treating a disease, especially if their treatment does not include pre-scription drugs, are in violation of the law and the FDA will close the doctors' office down. Why would the FDA create such a law? The only reason that makes any sense is that the FDA is out to protect the drug companies. This law is the reason why all labels on nutritional supplements have the disclaimer: This product is not intended to diagnose, treat, cure, or prevent any disease. The truth of the matter is many of these nutritional products do cure and prevent disease, but the supplement manufacturers are now forced to put this lie on their product labels because, if they don't, the FDA will close them down and throw them in jail. The FDA and their tactics to protect drug company profits are so blatant they remind me of how the Mafia goes about its business of protecting its profits. The only difference is the FDA is able to make up its own laws to allow it to operate within the law.

THE PATIENT'S NEW ROLE

So all of this begs the question: who protects you, the patient? As I said earlier, one of the reasons why I wanted to write this book is so that patients can learn to have a more proactive role in their cases. Right now they are not proactive. They go to their doctor and they just wait for the doctor to tell them what to do. If the doctor tells them to have invasive, radical surgery, most people will do it. But informed patients who understand how the system is set up and how it works don't have to be victims. They can make more informed decisions and choices and not rely solely on their medical doctors, who are more likely to provide options that are, unfortunately, not always best for their patients. Very often, doctors make decisions that are best for the doctors.

The biggest hurdle patients face in acting in their own best interests is knowledge. By reading this book you are going a long way toward overcoming this obstacle. To guide you, here are four simple steps to keep in mind as you read this book and as you come to a decision about which treatment to seek for your arthritis:

1. Understand that seeking Arthritis treatment from your medical doctor will result in only 4 possible treatments.
   1) drugs
   2) steroid shots
   3) physical therapy
   4) surgery

2. If none of these treatment options appeal to you, there is no need to seek help from your medical doctor. Now, you can focus on alternative treatment options.

3. If you do decide to have some form of medical treatment: make sure your doctor gets informed consent from you! Informed Consent is not only an ethical obligation, it is a legal requirement in all 50 states. Unfortunately just about all medical doctors don't do this. Here is a partial list of the things your treating doctor should discuss with you.
   1) what is your diagnosis
   2) what is the purpose of the proposed treatment
   3) what are the risks and benefits of the proposed treatment
   4) what are the alternative treatment options
   5) what are the risks and benefits of the alternatives

4. Whatever treatment you decide on, make sure to follow thru with the doctors recommendation. In my office, my recommendations are designed to give my patients the best possible chance to get better. Stopping care short of a doctors recommendation guarantees you will not achieve optimal results.

Also keep in mind: As you consider your options it is always best to start with treatments that are a lot less invasive and dangerous. Any type of injection or surgery should only be done when more conservative avenues have not worked. Not only does this make more sense because this mode of thinking is less risky, but it is also less expensive.

You will begin this process in the next chapter. You're going to learn more about arthritis, so you can better understand your current treatment options, including the particular one featured in this book. In the end it is my hope that you will be empowered to make an informed choice you can feel good about.

Chapter 2

A PRIMER ON YOUR ARTHRITIS

A rthritis occurs in many forms and affects men and women, young and old, in a variety of ways. As such, it is a complex condition. Perhaps that's why it can be difficult to treat. But the more you understand arthritis, the more informed you will be about making personal decisions about your level of treatment. We will start with the basics of arthritis in its most common form: osteoarthritis (OA)

If you take the literal Greek translation for the word osteoarthritis and break it down, you will have an accurate description of the condition:

osteo means "bone"
arthro means "joint"
itis means "inflammation"

Unfortunately, with OA, this definition is a bit of a misnomer because inflammation, while present in other types of arthritis such as rheumatoid arthritis, isn't really a primary symptom of OA. It may occur later on, secondarily or indirectly, but osteoarthritis first and foremost is a disease of the cartilage. I will explain this further on, but here, for your knowledge, is a brief rundown on the inflammatory types of arthritis:

INFLAMMATORY TYPES OF ARTHRITIS

- **Rheumatoid arthritis (RA)** is an autoimmune disease in which, for unknown reasons, the body attacks itself. With RA, specially, the immune system attacks the synovial lining of the joints of the body. The lining becomes inflamed and can progress until the joint is deformed. RA tends to strike the joints of the hands, feet, and elbows, but it can affect any joint in the body. The condition is marked by swollen, tender, and inflamed joints that become stiff and painful. The disease worsens over time, manifesting as "flare ups." RA tends to run in families and affect more women than men.

- **Systematic lupus erythematous (SLE)** is another autoimmune disease that attacks connective tissue. Common symptoms include joint pain, muscle ache, fatigue, and rash spread across the bridge of the nose and cheeks. Some people with this disorder may also be sensitive to light. For this reason laser therapy may not be indicated for some people with SLE. As this disease progresses, it may affect the heart, lungs, and kidneys, causing permanent damage.

- **Ankylosing spondylitis (AS):** This disease affects mostly young men. The tendons and ligaments of the spine become inflamed and make the spine stiff. The stiffness can get worse until the spine actually fuses itself together. On an X-ray, the spine of a patient with severe AS can look like a bamboo pole. The disease usually starts in the lower back and always involves the sacroiliac joints.

- **Psoriatic arthritis (PA):** People with the skin condition psoriasis can develop swollen and stiff joints. It affects the back most often and people with this condition have fingers and toes that look like "sausage digits." This condition affects men and women equally and the diagnosis of PA can be made when all of the following are present: red, scaly patches on the skin, pitted nails, and swollen joints.

I had recurring chronic pain in my knee, an age-related issue. I had trouble walking and could not run or squat. I thought I was becoming a candidate for knee replacement. Today, thanks to laser therapy, I can walk pain-free for miles and do light running. I'm looking forward to continuing healing.

Alan Dubinsky, age 59

- **Gout** is a metabolic disorder that renders the body unable to properly eliminate uric acid. The uric acid builds up to form crystals in the body, usually depositing in the big toe, but it can build up in any joint. Gout is characterized by red, swollen, and very painful joints. It primarily affects males who indulge in red meat, seafood, and alcoholic beverages. Gout was once considered the "rich man's disease" because only the rich could afford to indulge in such a diet. These days gout can be found in people of all economic classes. Like RA, it also tends to run in families.

THE OA DIFFERENCE

Notice how, with all the conditions described above, the joint is attacked directly and becomes inflamed almost immediately. That's why these conditions are inflammatory forms of arthritis. Osteoarthritis is different, however, in that the joint is not being attacked. Instead, a major, functioning piece of the joint, the "cartilage," is simply failing. This is the experience that most people who develop arthritis have. The cartilage is the bluish-white substance that is found on the end of bones. It is avascular, meaning it doesn't have any blood supply. However, cartilage is very important to the joints because its main function is to reduce friction and absorb force. The knee joint, for instance, is formed by the bottom of the femur (or thigh bone) and the top of the tibia (or shin bone). The edges of both bones are covered in cartilage, which has a very, very low friction coefficient; it is the lowest friction coefficient of any substance on the planet, so cartilage is very slippery. It enables the joint, or the two bones, to slide very easily around each other with very little friction. Cartilage is also quite rubbery and cushiony, so it can absorb the impact of walking or running.

The problem arises when, over time, cartilage begins to wear away. It will crack and break down, and that will cause the initial symptoms of arthritis, a feeling of stiffness in the joint. Those who are developing arthritis may notice they can't turn their neck as much or bend down as they used to. Or when they get up in the morning, their joints take 10 to 15 minutes to loosen up. The joints feel stiff and it may take a while to warm up and move freely again.

THE CONDITION PROGRESSES

As the condition progresses, and more and more cartilage breaks down, the sufferer feels more pain. At first, the pain might not be very severe, just a kind of ache that can usually be relieved with rest but is exacerbated with activity such as walking and running. The more the cartilage breaks down, the more severe the symptoms become. The dull pain can become sharp pain, and the sharp pain that was once relieved with rest remains painful whether the sufferer rests or not. In the worst cases arthritis sufferers develop a visible deformity in the joint.

Finally, the joint will deteriorate to the point where the cartilage is virtually nonexistent. Once the cartilage is gone, the actual bone will ache a lot more as the force and the friction increases. Then the bones themselves, especially at the end of the joint, begin to break down and become sclerotic or very hard. On an X-ray, the cortical (outside edge of a bone) that is sclerotic looks very, very white. It's actually very easy to diagnose osteoarthritis by looking at an X-ray, especially one of the knee, because it is a very big joint. You can clearly see the bone hardening; you see the extra white, thick end of the bone, and the space between the bones, where there is supposed to be fluid and cartilage, is virtually gone. The bones just sit directly on top of each other, "bone on bone."

As a side note: you can't see the cartilage on an X-ray. You can see the joint space and other things, but if you really want to know the extent of the cartilage damage, you would have to get a magnetic resonance image, better known as an MRI, which allows you to see more of the soft tissue or cartilage in the joint. There are some cost restrictions with MRIs—they are expensive. However, getting a clear picture of the extent of the damage in the cartilage is not necessary unless you are undergoing a scientific study and doing a before-and-after study to determine if a treatment has influenced the rebuilding of cartilage. Other than that, X-rays are the preferred method of imaging. Remember, OA is not an inflammatory arthritis, such as rheumatoid arthritis, or systematic lupus erythematous. An inflammatory type of arthritis means the condition is more systemic and the inflammation is a direct consequence of the disease or type of arthritis. However, with OA, the inflammation is simply a by-product of the loss of cartilage, the true marker of OA. Once the cartilage breaks down, the resulting friction and force on the joint leads to the inflammation. So indirectly, OA will cause inflammation, but it's not a direct consequence of the arthritis.

OA OR RA?

Osteoarthritis mainly affects the weight-bearing joints of the body: the knees, the hips, the spine. It also affects the hands, the wrist, the shoulders, and the feet. In examining a patient with arthritic symptoms, there are several markers to look for to help diagnose OA as opposed to RA. OA primarily affects distal interphalangeal (DIP) joints. These are the joints located closest to the fingernails. They are called Heberden's nodes. The type of joint that's closest to the knuckle, or in the middle of the finger, is known as a PIP joint (proximal interphalangeal joint—Bouchard's nodes). These joints are more affected by rheumatoid arthritis. In terms of progression, OA usually affects one side of the body first: it will develop in one knee and then the other knee, or in one hand and then the other hand. RA, however, affects the body symmetrically and simultaneously. Both hands will be affected, or both knees and both elbows.

WHO GETS ARTHRITIS?

One in three adults will have, or be diagnosed with, arthritis in his or her lifetime. Some 60 percent of people over the age of 65 will have OA and unfortunately, that number is expected to climb as time goes by. In fact, it is expected to double by 2030. Why is the rate of incidence growing so quickly? The answer is in the risk factor for OA, and there really is just one: being overweight or obese. While OA does tend to run in families, the big trend in the United States is that more and more people are overweight and that number has been climbing steadily throughout the years. There's a direct link between obesity rates and osteoarthritis: the heavier you are, the more stressors you place on your joints. Eventually your joints will wear down a lot faster than those of someone who is of normal weight or ideal weight.

AGE AND ARTHRITIS

Because of our limited knowledge about arthritis, we, as a society, tend to see arthritis as a condition of the elderly. But that's not always the case. Developing arthritis, heredity aside, is more a function of how the body has been maintained and how it is used. For instance, a man who has been in several motor vehicle accidents, causing trauma and damage to his joints, is almost guaranteed to develop OA later in life. On the other hand, someone who goes through life with no major accidents or broken bones is a lot less likely to develop OA later in life. In general, those aged 45 and younger who develop arthritis are more likely to be men, but once we hit age 55, arthritis is seen more in women. Women are twice as likely as men to develop arthritis when they are 55 or older.

THE TWO SIDES OF OA

This discussion of age is good time to make this point about osteo-arthritis: it comes in two forms: primary and secondary. How these forms manifest depends on the patient's age and activity levels. Primary OA is seen mostly in people over the age of 45. This is the type of OA that progresses slowly, as I described above. You first get the stiffness that pro-gresses and worsens and affects weight-bearing joints such as the knees and the hips. Secondary osteoarthritis is different because the arthritis is secondary to some other form of trauma the patient has experienced. A good example would be a football player or any type of athlete who once broke an ankle, or severely injured a limb while playing sports. Ten years later that athlete will have arthritis, not because the joint has worn down over time but because of the severe trauma of the original injury. This isn't limited to athletes. Those who work with their hands, such as auto mechanics, are also more likely to develop arthritis in their hands a lot earlier than those who don't work with their hands. Secondary OA progresses much more quickly than primary OA. Someone who has secondary arthritis probably developed it a lot earlier in life than someone who didn't have any type of trauma or injury.

> Laser treatment relieved 85 percent of the pain on lower back, hip, thigh, and right leg. I can still drive and I'm able to walk longer. I can do yard work. I can sleep better too. My wife and I went back to ballroom dancing. No jitterbug, swing dancing, no high tech dancing, but we can dance the rumba, cha-cha, meringue, fox trot, and waltz.
>
> **—Antone Fernandez, age 85**

PREVENTION

Is it possible to prevent osteoarthritis? When you consider certain risk factors are under our control—weight control and healthy habits—you would think that it is possible. However, a lot of people, physicians included, tend to think arthritis is inevitable—that no matter what you do, you're going to have OA as you get older. They think arthritis is simply a disease of aging, but it's more complicated than that. When people experience no trauma in their lifetime, meaning they never had any major accidents, or broken bones, and they took good care of their bodies by exercising, stretching, and eating a proper diet, their chances of developing arthritis are very low compared to those who experience a lot of traumas, have a bad diet, and do not exercise. So even though the medical community perceives arthritis to be inevitable, as you can see here, it is not that cut-and-dried. OA is a progressive condition, so the more time that passes, the more damage can be done to the cartilage. Anyone who is 80 or 90 years old has some arthritis, but those who take good care of their bodies and who experience only minor traumas will have minimal arthritis and the pain is not likely to be significant or disabling. You are not going to be completely free of arthritis if you live a long life, but you definitely can control the extent of the damage and limit the chances that your arthritis will significantly diminish your quality of life. A great example of someone who had a healthy lifestyle and lived a long, active life without arthritis would be Jack Lalanne. He is known as the pioneer of physical fitness. He spent his entire life eating healthy food and working out before any of the benefits of exercise were published or hypothesized. He lived to be 96 years old and was active until his final years. When he was 70 he was shackled to 70 boats and he towed them a mile and a half across Long Beach harbor.

TREATING OA

The conventional medical community also believes that OA is incurable—once you have it, you're going to have to live with it. There's nothing you can do about it. If you follow the treatment that your conventional physician recommends, it becomes something of a self-fulfilling prophecy: the arthritis isn't curable because conventional medical treatments don't cure anything and they are not meant to cure anything. Unfortunately, when patients go to their doctor, and that's usually what they do first, no matter what kind of pain or problem they have, the doctor's primary response is, "You're getting old; you just have to live with it." If the pain gets too bad, your doctor may recommend you take Advil or Aleve, but for the most part he or she will tell you to live with it for the rest of your life. I think this is terrible advice and it's misleading because the class-4 laser offers patients with severe, chronic arthritis pain long-term relief. It is an absolute shame to think there are millions of people across the country suffering from arthritis pain, and they continue to suffer because conventional medical doctors are not aware or are not willing to refer their arthritic patients to class-4 laser therapists.

That's why I wanted to put this book together: so you can understand the nature of arthritis and all of the available treatment options. Treatment for arthritis has not changed for decades. A patient with

> When I first came to Dr. Alosa I could not raise my right arm. It was so painful to brush my hair and to apply my contact lens. After receiving several laser treatments, the pain is gone and I can lift and do everything again with my right arm! I am a private housekeeper, thus I need the use of my right arm to do my work. After laser treatments, I am as good as new, so I can continue my occupation as a housekeeper.
>
> **—Betty Ann Lee, age 75**

OA now will get the same exact treatment options as in the 1980s, with the exception of joint replacement surgery. Laser technology has improved the prognosis for anyone with any type of arthritis, but the prognosis for a patient in the conventional medical model has not changed in decades. Conventional medicine is stuck in the same thinking that has plagued it for years—namely, that every patient who seeks relief can only be treated with drugs or surgery. All those suffering from arthritis must take responsibility for their treatment and try class-4 laser therapy. Every day that they procrastinate is another day they have to live in pain and refrain from doing things they enjoy, such as playing with their grandkids, golfing, tennis, or working in the garden.

Dr. Alosa,

Thank you for bringing LiteCure deep-tissue laser treatments to Hawaii and to my daughter who saw your ad in the newspaper and called it to my attention. We both took advantage of getting our first evaluation.

After my first treatment for my sciatic problem, I felt 80 percent better and after each treatment, it gets better and better. I am now walking a little longer and able to do more work in my yard.

This laser treatment is done with no pain; I just love the warm sensation surrounding the affected area and shoots all the way down my legs; it's wonderful! I have recommended this to my family and friends and hope they will try it.

With much aloha,
Betty Inoue, age 77

TIMING OF TREATMENT

Arthritis is a progressive condition that gets worse over time. Generally speaking, the longer someone has had arthritis, the longer it will take to fix it, costing more money and more time. There is one caveat to this: if the arthritis has advanced to the stage where the joint is visibly enlarged and deformed, no treatment can change that deformity. Once the calcium has built up and the bone has hyper-trophied, you develop bone spurs in the joint. Once the damage is done, there is no treatment that can reverse that damage. This occurs mostly in the fingers and I have had many patients ask me if the laser can help with the visible deformity. Unfortunately, there is nothing that can be done to remove that damage. I can give an example of surgeons trying to remove bone spurs in the knee joint, which has been proven scientifically to provide no benefit to patients. This involves arthroscopic surgery, in which a surgeon will go in and make three small incisions around the knee. Then the surgeon goes in and scopes it, which means he or she will just scrape away some of the bony overgrowth. This treatment, unfortunately, usually causes more problems and exacerbates the arthritis. It causes trauma to the joint, which causes arthritis! The joint often will become inflamed and develop scar tissue. Many times I have seen patients who have severe arthritis of the knee. Almost all of them have had arthroscopic surgery, and they're pretty shocked when I tell them that the surgery probably either caused their arthritis or made it worse. They felt better right after the surgery only to have their condition get much worse soon after.

While laser treatment cannot change the appearance of a deformed joint, it can help immensely with the pain and stiffness you feel. In my office we have, many times, helped patients who have been severely arthritic, even disabled, for extended periods of time. I had one patient who had been disabled since the 1970s, due to a major car accident. His X-rays were among the worst I have ever seen as far as the degeneration in his lower back. But after the treatments in my office, he no longer needed to use a cane. He was able to walk his dogs again and work in his garden. The treatment totally changed his life.

This testimony is from someone who had tried every type of medical intervention to no avail. But after 20 treatments with the laser, he was pain-free because of the power of the laser. In my professional experience there is no case that is too bad or too severe: we have seen some of the worst cases in my office and we have been able to help these patients get better. It's as simple as that.

THE COST OF ARTHRITIS

Arthritis is the number-one cause of chronic pain and disability in the United States. It accounts for 17 percent of all disability in the country. But consider that statistic in this context: heart disease is the number-one cause of death in the United States, but it accounts for just 11 percent of all the disability here. That should give you an idea of how chronic arthritis is. Now here's an idea of how prevalent it is: Cancer affects one in three adults in the United States and is the second leading cause of death. The incidence rate for arthritis is exactly the same: one in three. That means if you've ever known someone who has developed cancer in his or her lifetime, you will also know someone with arthritis. That's

> I have suffered lower back pain and subsequent problems with sciatica and leg problems for forty years, all stemming from an auto accident in 1970. After the very first laser treatment I noticed marked improvement in my pain level and have progressively improved as if from a miracle! After treatments I feel like I've had an 85 percent improvement and can now walk without a cane! I look forward to my next appointments because the treatments WORK! I am already almost pain free and can sleep thru the night. My quality of life has improved exponentially.
>
> **—Kenneth Kawaguchi**

how common arthritis is, and unfortunately, the rate of occurrence is only increasing, not decreasing. I believe the most popular treatments, which involve injections, drugs, or surgery, are adding to the problem.

And arthritis is an expensive ailment. Whether we realize it or not, we are all paying for the high incidence of arthritis in this country. Consider these numbers: Arthritis results in $15 billion of direct medical costs billed from 44 million outpatient visits and 750,000 hospitalizations a year. If you include the cost to society of lost work productivity, the price of arthritis goes up to $83 billion a year. That's every single year, just for arthritis! I don't know about you, but I think that is a pretty powerful statement.

So if arthritis is the number-one cause of chronic pain, and it is costing all this money, you would think finding an effective treatment for it would be very important.

> I'm relieved of pain and tightness I get in my neck and shoulders after working at the office and on the computer. With the heat and deep penetration, neck and shoulders felt relaxed, loose and no more tightness. The results were good, plus I'm very satisfied and would do this again when necessary. I don't have the feeling of the pain and tightness every day. I don't have to do daily stretches, apply heat, use massage items to relieve pain/tightness. It also helped ease minor numbness from pinched nerves from several years ago.
>
> —**Blanche Kinoshita, 62**

THE COST, FINANCIALLY AND PHYSICALLY, OF CURRENT TREATMENTS

These days a patient diagnosed with arthritis will most likely be treated with one of the following:

- prescription medications or over-the-counter medications meant to control inflammation
- injections that involve shooting a joint with corticosteroids or epidurals

Let's look at surgery first. It is by far the most expensive arthritis treatment done today. The cost of a spinal fusion surgery can run from $50,000 to $80,000, not including the cost of outpatient visits for rehabilitation and follow up. Unfortunately, even with all the cost and risk associated with surgery, patients often don't get very good results from these procedures. As I mentioned earlier, many patients don't get any better—they often get worse and incur more medical expenses because they have to keep going back to the doctor. Also, a lot of times, one surgery leads to two, or even three surgeries. You can see how these costs can escalate out of control and contribute to the major problems we have now in our health-care system. The surgeries performed for arthritis are usually one of these three procedures: spinal surgery, knee replacement surgery (TKR), and hip replacement surgery (THR).

SPINAL SURGERY

Any type of spinal surgery will usually target the neck or lower back. Arthritis in any of those two areas of the spine can create very strong symptoms down the arms—if the arthritis is in the neck—or down the legs if it is in the lower back. That's because all the nerves that supply your shoulder all the way down to your arms, hands, and fingers come from the cervical spine in the neck. The same thing goes for the lower back: all the nerves that go down to your legs all the way to your toes, exit in the lower back. When doctors perform spinal surgery in these areas, they are doing a laminectomy or a hemilaminectomy or generally known as decompression surgery. The lamina is part of the vertebrae that connects the vertebral body to the posterior elements of the vertebrae.

This means they cut off the posterior aspect of the spine. The rationale is that the nerves of the spinal cord are being pinched against this part of the spine. The surgeons figure that removing the entire back portion of the spine will fix the problem because the nerves will have nothing to press up against, hence the term decompression.

> At the beginning of the year, I started to notice a persistent throbbing at the base of both thumbs. As a professional musician, I need to have full use of both hands, so I began to get very worried. The discomfort was most pronounced in the left thumb, which I use constantly. Whenever I moved it, the throbbing would turn to pain. I would be thinking about it at all times during concerts and practice sessions. Regular massaging of the tender areas did not bring much relief. What could I do? I definitely did not want to risk the surgery and I knew that cortisone shots would only give temporary relief.
>
> When I saw Dr. Alosa's ad, I decided to give his treatment a try. After just several sessions, I noticed the pain was less constant. Gradually, it went away entirely. Now, I can focus my complete attention on playing and not worry about the pain. Thank you, Dr. Alosa, and Staff!
>
> **—Robert Larm, age 54**

When a spinal joint becomes arthritic, it gets bigger from bony overgrowth, called bone spurs. Because this bone is growing out and then pushing the nerves of the spinal cord up against the back of the spine, surgeons reason that if they cut the back of the spine out, the nerves will have more room when the arthritis pushes them back. So the surgeons cut the back part of the spine off and remove the bony structures. This is great because the nerves have nothing to push against anymore. However, the process destabilizes the area to a great extent, and that destabilization will cause more arthritis. The body is trying to support the structure and keep it from being unstable. But the arthritis actually accelerates because there's so much more pressure on the joint, and the body has only half of that spinal segment to deal with all the weight and stress of the body.

The stress causes the area to wear out a lot faster. This will often lead doctors to do a spinal fusion, either in tandem with a laminectomy or down the road because the area remains so unstable they must put in pins to fuse the spine together. So in essence, they are mutilating the human spine in the effort to cure the arthritis, which makes absolutely no sense. Here's another head turning fact: spinal fusion surgery has a *1 in 100* success rate. That's just 1 percent. This information was published in 1994 by the U.S. Public Health Service Agency for Health Care Policy and Research (AHCPR). I don't know about you, but I'm not allowing anyone to cut my spine open for a very risky surgery with a 1 percent success rate.

But this low success rate should not be a surprise. The spine has 24 movable bones for a reason: all 24 of those bones are meant to move on each other and work as one in a long, schematic chain. Fusing two or three of the segments together changes the biomechanics of the spine and creates more load and stress on the non-fused segments. This will then cause more arthritis and more pain. I have many patients who have already had surgery, once, twice, or even three times, and they have chronic, life-altering pain because the damage that was done to the spine is permanent. You simply cannot cut out part of the spine, put screws in it, and then expect this process to fix the problem and not cause other types of problems. It reminds me of one of the very first medical procedures done in history: trepanning. Trepanning is when doctors cut a hole in the patient's skull to allow the "bad spirits" out. I would like to think modern medicine has come a long way since then, but unfortunately doctors doing spinal surgery are still mutilating the body in an attempt to heal it. That is why surgery should always be considered a treatment of last resort, done only when every other treatment has been tried and found unsuccessful. Furthermore, spinal surgery is almost never an emergency procedure. For 99 percent of patients, it is an elective procedure just like cosmetic surgery. This puts the power in the patients' hands; it is 100 percent up to them to decide if they want to undergo a spinal procedure. Please, don't let a surgeon coerce you into anything you are not comfortable with because once the surgery is done, there is no going back.

For those patients who are reading this book and have already had a surgical procedure performed on their spine, there is good news: my laser has the ability to remodel scar tissue into healthy elastic tissue again through a process called angiogenesis. Angiogenesis is the formation of new blood capillaries and vessels. I have treated hundreds of patients with failed back surgery syndrome and most have gotten pain relief; some have had profound, life-changing responses.

Arthroscopic surgery is a less invasive surgical procedure because it involves three small incisions in the skin and is conducted with the aid of an arthroscope. The arthroscope is guided by a lighted scope attached to a TV monitor so the surgeon can observe the joint from the inside. This type of surgery is often used on the knee joint to treat symptoms associated with OA by removing pieces of cartilage, repairing or removing a meniscus or to smooth aged, worn-out cartilage. But arthroscopic surgery can be used on other joints as well, such as the shoulder.

However, this form of treatment is not a very effective option for OA sufferers. In fact, a study was carried out in which patients were divided into three groups of subjects. One group received debridement treatment (cutting off pieces of cartilage); the second group received lavage (flushing the joint out with fluid, irrigation); and the last group had incisions made but no procedure was done. All three groups reported just about the same results: each had slightly less pain, but as time went on, the nonprocedure group actually had the best results. This only highlighted the real problem with this type of surgery: it actually causes arthritis. As I mentioned earlier, anytime you cut into a joint and scrape, cut, or file the joint surface, you are traumatizing the joint just as you would if you were in a motor vehicle accident and

After my years of playing football, basketball, and racquetball, I was a prime candidate for knee replacement. I had no cartilage in my left knee. I decided to try class-4, deep-tissue laser treatment as a last resort before knee replacement surgery. At first, I did not feel any new changes until the fifth treatment. The pain in my knee started to subside. I could fall asleep without an ice pack on my knee. Dr. Alosa recommended eight weeks of treatment, two treatments twice a week. As a result of the treatment, I can walk longer distances without pain and sleep with no pain. This is not a 100 percent cure. However, I feel 70 percent to 80 percent better than I did without the treatments.

—Manny Rezentes, age 73

broke your leg. Who would choose to do that, especially when science proves arthroscopic knee surgery doesn't work?

On July 11, 2002, the *New England Journal of Medicine* published a landmark study titled, "A Controlled Trial of Arthroscopic Surgery for Osteoarthritis of the Knee." This study was done extremely well. It involved a large group of patients; it was double blinded; and participants were randomly placed. The patients were randomly placed in two groups and both the patients and the doctors conducting the study did not know which group they were in (double blind). One group received an actual arthroscopic procedure and the other group had the small incisions made, but no arthroscopic procedure was done. The patients were followed for 24 months and the results shocked the medical community. The results showed no difference between the two groups. The patients who had the sham procedure done experienced the same results as the group who had the actual procedure done! Ladies and gentlemen, this is all you need to know from this point forward about arthroscopic knee surgery. It does not work and demonstrates what drives modern medicine because it is still being performed today when science says it doesn't work.

Total knee replacement (TKR) surgery is a treatment option for the severely damaged knee. During knee replacement surgery the surgeon cuts away the damaged bone and cartilage from the femur (thigh bone), tibia (shin bone), and knee cap and replaces it with an artificial joint made of metal alloys or high-grade plastics. There are several things patients need to consider when making a decision about undergoing (TKR). Possible side effects can include:

- knee stiffness
- infection
- blood clots
- heart attack
- stroke
- nerve damage

Also, anyone under the age of 55 should not undergo TKR because the artificial parts have a limited life span. As of today a TKR may be good for only 10 to 15 years maximum before the artificial knee will have to be replaced. That means those in their 40s, receiving an artificial knee, would automatically have to have more surgery in their 50s—not an ideal situation. Surgery can be very painful, and for TKR in particular, the rehabilitation process is long and arduous and can take up to twelve months.

Asking patients to undergo more than one TKR on the same knee is asking a lot, considering all the risks and the long and painful rehabilitation. Add to this the fact that patients can expect diminished returns with each surgery. In other words, replacing an artificial joint has a lower success rate, due to increased risks and scar tissue formation. With so much to consider, the decision of whether or not to have a TKR is naturally a tough one for people to make. Here are some guidelines, courtesy of the Mayo Clinic, to think about before making a decision to undergo this surgery:

- You pain is severe and disabling. The pain should be to the point where it is difficult for you to perform simple tasks such as walking. It should also be constant and unremitting.
- You have tried all other available options.
- You are 55 years of age or older.
- Your health is good. You are not obese or diabetic.

TOTAL HIP REPLACEMENT (THR)

Hip replacement surgery carries with it a lot of the same risks as TKR, so I won't repeat those again. However, I would like to discuss one particular risk associated with hip replacements. Sometimes the prosthesis can loosen over time, causing pain and requiring more surgery to fix it. Another problem can arise when the surgeon doesn't cut the femur to exactly the correct length. A patient may end up with one leg longer than the other, and the greater the leg length discrepancy, the greater the side effects. Some of these effects include back and hip pain because every time a patient walks, the uneven stress on one leg will be compensated for in other parts of the body. This also leads to pain and joint problems in other parts of the body such as the lumbar spine or sacroiliac joints. Can you imagine going through the rigors of surgery and rehabilitation only to be told you have to repeat the entire process again? I have seen what that can do to a patient's quality of life. I had a patient come to me in 2011 with severe hip pain. Upon taking her health history, I found out she had undergone four surgeries on her left hip! Her first hip replacement didn't fit properly so they had to replace it with another one. Then that replacement was slipping and causing considerable pain, so the surgeon had to operate again on the same hip to stop it from slipping. Then they had to go in two more times to tighten her hip.

After these four separate surgeries on her left hip, this poor woman was still in considerable, unremitting pain. As you can imagine, this turned her life upside down. She could barely walk. Sitting for long periods was difficult, and she couldn't play with her grandkids. Her pain was so bad it would keep her up at night, so she couldn't get adequate rest. All told, her health had really deteriorated since she first agreed to the surgery. Thankfully my laser treatments were able to get her some pain relief.

INJECTIONS AND PRESCRIPTION DRUGS

If you are being treated for your arthritis by a medical doctor, chances are you are receiving cortisone injections or prescription drugs. First, here's an important point you need to know: All medical treatments are palliative. This means that the doctor knows your condition cannot be cured or fixed permanently so the goal is just to do things to alleviate the pain temporarily. In fact, none of the drugs that doctors prescribe are meant to fix or cure anything. They are just meant to alleviate some of the symptoms associated with the arthritis. Unfortunately, the drugs are just masking the symptoms while the problem or disease continues to deteriorate. The patient is actually getting worse but doesn't realize it because he or she can't feel it. Over time, the disease only progresses even further. The same goes for injections: the shots are just meant to temporarily alleviate some of the pain. The commonest thing doctors use in this instance is cortisone, a kind of steroid, or corticosteroid, that is also an anti-inflammatory. Sometimes the injection works; sometimes it doesn't. I've had patients who felt no change whatsoever. I've had patients who say their pain had been relieved for extended periods of time. The pain relief may last a few months or if you are lucky, a year or more. But no matter how long you get relief, one thing is certain: the pain will come back. It is just a matter of when it will return. Due to the dangerous side effects of steroid injections, they should not be done more than three times a year. Another problem with these shots is that they tend to have diminished returns, meaning subsequent injections should not be expected to get the same amount of relief as the first. One last thing to know is that these injections usually hurt like hell.

The side effects of corticosteroids should not be taken lightly because they have the ability to suppress your immune system. Your immune system is the only thing that protects you day in and day out from deadly bacteria and viruses. Steroids can cause cancer! Your immune system is not the only thing that becomes suppressed: the adrenal glands also become suppressed, which leads to weight gain. On top of that, you can expect to have weakened bones or osteo-porosis from cortisone use. So your weakened bones will have to carry more weight, which will make you a prime candidate for bone fractures.

Let me give you an example of what continued steroid use can do to your bones. I had a patient who was asthmatic and had been taking steroids for a long time. She was walking in her house, tripped on the carpet, and fell on her arm. Her humerus bone in her upper arm didn't just break – it shattered into many pieces. Under normal circumstances a fall of that nature would not even create a fracture, but because of her steroid use, the bone fragmented. These are some of the risks you take when you choose cortisone injections.

The clinical introduction of corticosteroids began in 1949. It is postulated that corticosteroids reduce inflammation by inhibiting either the synthesis or the release of a number of proinflammatory substances (prostaglandin and arachidonic acid) and by causing a reversible anesthetic effect. When researching the mechanism of action for corticosteroids, you will notice a lot words such as *postulated, unknown, uncertain,* and *complex.* These words indicate that scientists do not truly understand how these steroid injections produce their anti-inflammatory effects. This is not unusual. In fact, the more time you spend looking at the available research for many of the most common medical procedures done in this country, the more you will realize there is shockingly little research and understanding of how most medical procedures work.

UNSETTLING STATISTICS

Some 106,000 deaths occur every year because of the nonerror, adverse effects of prescription drugs. This is an important point for you to understand, so let me reiterate: over 100,000 patients are dying every year from drugs that are properly prescribed to them. In other words, the doctor gave the right drug to the right patient in the right dose and the patient still died. This clearly demonstrates the inherent danger in taking prescription drugs because no one ever knows in advance how any person will react to a certain drug. Some may be fine while others will abruptly drop dead without warning! This is because humans are all biologically different from each other, thus making it impossible to know for sure how someone will react to a certain drug. This problem is made much worse by the FDA's often rushed, abbreviated, drug-approval process.

Aspirin, for instance, has got to be one of the most widely used drugs in the country and yet no one knows how aspirin works as an antipyretic (lowers fever). I could go on and on with examples like this because according to Dr. David Eddy and his research in the *British Medical Journal* (1991 303:798), only 15 percent of medical interventions are supported by scientific evidence. This is partly because only 1 percent of articles in medical journals are scientifically sound.

Since we are discussing aspirin, this would be a good time to discuss other common anti-inflammatory drugs, both prescription and over-the-counter. Since most arthritis patients begin their treatment with some sort of drug therapy, it would be helpful to understand how these drugs work and their possible side effects. Once informed, the patient can make the determination if drug therapy is a viable option.

NSAIDS

Nonsteroidal anti-inflammatory drugs (NSAIDs) work by blocking the production of prostaglandin, a hormone-like substance in the body that causes pain and inflammation. Side effects include high blood pressure, ulcers, nausea, cramps, diarrhea, constipation, nervousness, confusion, heart attack, swelling fingers/hands/feet, weight gain, and anaphylaxis.

Note that anaphylaxis is a severe allergic reaction that creates difficulty in breathing, dizziness, fainting, and an increased heart rate. This is a medical emergency. If you ever experience any of these symptoms call 911 right away.

I think the public believes drugs that are sold over the counter are generally safe. Because the public's perception of these drugs is that they are safe, people don't take the proper precautions that they do when taking a prescription drug. According to Dr. Frank Hamilton, MD, NSAIDs account for 20,000 deaths and up to 200,000 hospitalizations every year!

THE NEW NSAID: COX-2 INHIBITOR

As I mentioned earlier in this book, Vioxx was approved by the FDA in 1999 and it was promoted as the new and improved anti-inflammatory without serious gastrointestinal complications. However, from the start, the makers of Vioxx and Celebrex had deceived the public. During the approval process with the FDA, the data these companies reported to the FDA was not the same as was published. This is not new. When drug companies fund their own research, the companies always seem to show their product is better than the competition. It has been proven time and time again that there is widespread publication bias in the research community, resulting in dangerous, overpriced drugs coming to market that are no better than drugs already on the market. As it turned out, the Cox-2 drugs did not help protect the stomach lining. In fact, they were just as likely to cause bleeding as the other class of NSAIDs.

Merck eventually had to pull its drug off the market when a large amount of research revealed a much higher rate of heart attack in Vioxx users. One study, published in *The Lancet* medical journal in October 2002, showed that Vioxx had caused 88,000 deaths and 140,000 cases of heart disease. Obviously, new does not equal better.

OVER-THE-COUNTER DRUGS

Acetaminophen (Tylenol) is an analgesic (pain reliever) and anti-pyretic (reduces fever).

NSAIDs (aspirin, ibuprophen, Advil, Motrin) are analgesic, antipyretic, and anti-inflammatory drugs.

Potential NSAIDs problems and side effects include irritation of the stomach lining. Even short-term use can cause stomach irritation, gastritis, and ulcers. These drugs, even though bought over the counter, are still life threatening because an ulcer can cause internal bleeding, which can cause death. Obviously, any internal bleeding is dangerous, but only one out of five people who have a serious gastrointestinal complication will have any warning signs. This becomes even more serious when patients are also taking blood thinners, such as Plavix or Warfarin, because these drugs don't allow blood to coagulate. Patients who are on any type of blood-thinning drug are even more at risk from serious GI complications. NSAIDs (with the exception of aspirin) raise blood pressure. High blood pressure is known as the silent killer because it has no symptoms. High blood pressure leads to increased incidents of stroke, kidney disease, and heart disease.

Acetaminophen is the number-one cause of liver failure. In fact, acetaminophen accounts for more liver failure than all other drugs combined. Potential side effects include stomach bleeding, and the drug is estimated to cause 5,000 cases of kidney failure every year. Acetaminophen is found in a lot of other over-the-counter medications, so patients may be unaware of how much they are actually consuming, which can lead to overdosing and the serious complications that come with that. In 2002 an FDA panel found acetaminophen was involved in 56,680 emergency room visits, 26,000 hospitalizations and about 450 deaths a year. People who use acetaminophen on a daily basis over a long period of time are at an increased risk of kidney failure.

SHOULD YOU TAKE ACETAMINOPHEN?

Only one in three people get pain reduction of 20 percent or more using a maximum dose of 4,000 mg/day. At doses of about 2,000 mg, acetaminophen may cause stomach bleeding and more serious complications. If only 2,000 mg has the potential to cause side effects, by doubling the dose, you are basically doubling your chances of incurring side effects. I don't want to risk death for the minimal, temporary relief associated with acetaminophen. If this drug had the potential to permanently cure arthritis pain, maybe it would be worth the risk to take it, but since I'd have to take it every day for minimal relief, I think acetaminophen, or any other drug used as the prime method of treatment for osteoarthritis, is very limited and not worth the risks.

Let's go back to an earlier statistic: only 15 percent of medical treatments are supported by science, yet medical doctors and the general public perceive medicine as a superior choice of treatment compared to other types of health care because medicine is scientifically based and the others are not. But none of these medical treatments for arthritis are meant to provide any type of long-term pain relief—none! They are just temporary palliatives at best. That's what makes the laser so remarkable: it does provide long-term pain relief without the dangerous side effects and risks of injections or drugs. In the next chapter we'll learn more about lasers and find out exactly how they do what they do.

Chapter 3

THE HEALING POWER OF LASERS

As a society we have known and used lasers for years. Everyone is probably more familiar with the lasers we see in the checkout line at the grocery story or the lasers that scan a book when you check it out from the library. We see laser pointers during a PowerPoint presentation and we know Lasik eye surgery involves some sort of laser. But what exactly is a laser and how does it work?

DECODING THE TERM

The word *laser* is actually an acronym for Light Amplification Stimulated Emission of Radiation. What's important to note here is that the radiation is nonionizing radiation. Unlike X-rays and gamma rays that can cause cancer and other detrimental effects, the laser's type of radiation is safe. The acronym *LASER* also explains what a laser really does: it uses amplified light, which stimulates the emission of radiation, which starts the healing process in the body. That's pretty much how the laser works in a nutshell. But the first thing that comes to mind when someone talks about lasers is that they don't really know much about the technology; they think it's a new technology. Actually this type of technology has been around for over 40 years. A very low-level laser was first used in experiments back in the late 1960s by a scientist named Andre Mester. He noticed that laser energy was causing cellular changes in mice. This was over 40 years ago. Since then there have been over 2500 studies done on laser therapy and they have shown that the laser actually can stimulate the body to heal itself through cellular repair and cellular regeneration. The type of laser that I use to treat patients is relatively new—it was cleared by the FDA in 2003. But the research behind laser therapy has been some 40 years in the making.

The LASIK eye surgery, which involves using a laser to reshape the surface of the eye, was revolutionary when it first came out. That particular laser therapy revolutionized the treatment of vision problems. Now, 15 watt, class-4 laser therapy is revolutionizing the treatment of arthritis. We also have surgical lasers that are able to perform procedures that could not have been done traditionally using a scalpel. With the laser, it is possible to perform very precise types of surgery that wouldn't have been possible before the laser's invention.

COLD LASERS

The laser I use in my office is a Lightforce class-4, deep-tissue laser. It is a dual diode laser with 15 watts of power on continuous wave (CW) with 900 J (joules) of energy delivered per minute. It is also called a cold laser, which is a misnomer because this laser actually produces warmth that patients can feel during treatment. Here's a little history that I hope can clear up the confusion caused by the cold laser's name. Back in 1967, when scientists were first theorizing what lasers could do, they observed how the laser caused cellular changes in mice but also created heat. Many skeptics claimed that the cellular changes were caused by heat and not light from the laser. So the scientists measured the temperature changes during the study and they found them to be insignificant, proving it was the laser light that was making the cellular changes and not the heat from the laser. The *cold laser* term has stuck because of those initial studies. Patients' confusion seems to remain, however, because the cellular activity caused by the laser is a photochemical response to the light, not a photothermal response. But some patients still believe the heat is therapeutic because they can feel it, and they are often surprised when I tell them it's the light that's causing the changes. Adding to the confusion is the fact that patients can feel warmth when treated with a class-4 laser but no temperature change when treated with a lower-class of laser such as class 3. Nevertheless, all lasers, aside from surgical lasers, are called *cold lasers*.

THE LASER CLASSIFICATION SYSTEM

All lasers are classified by the manufacturer and labeled with the appropriate warning labels. They use the following criteria to classify the lasers: wavelength, average power, total energy per pulse. There are currently two classification systems in use. One is based on the FDA laser in existence prior to 2002, and the other one is based on the standard governing the safety of lasers internationally (IEC), which was substantially revised in 2001, when the classification system was also modified. Three new laser classes (1m, 2m, 3R) were created and class 3a was removed.

Simply put, the classes are derived from the laser's power. The lowest level is class 1. These are the lasers you see in the grocery store, and PowerPoint lasers. The levels of power go up to 4. The class-4 level includes lasers used in an office setting like mine where musculoskeletal injuries are treated. Beyond that are the surgical lasers, such as a CO2 class laser, which can ablate or cut tissue.

Warning: For all those readers who are not doctors or scientists, in the following pages I will explain how the laser works. I will use words I'm sure many of you have never heard of, but I think it is very important to explain how the laser works because it is a question I get all the time from my patients. I will do my best to use layman terms when possible, but I have to include the scientific explanations for readers who are doctors and scientists.

THE CLASS–4 LASER AND ARTHRITIS TREATMENT

The class-4 laser has a power of 15 watts. In comparison, a class-3 laser has only 500 mw of power at the most. Power affects penetration, dosage, and treatment time. More power offers deeper penetration, higher therapeutic dosages, and decreased treatment times. This makes the class-4 laser very effective in treating arthritis and musculoskeletal problems affecting deeper anatomical structures such as the spine or the hip. The lower-powered lasers aren't really effective because they don't have the power to allow the photons in the laser to travel deep enough into the body to hit the target tissues, and you cannot make up for insufficient power by increasing treatment time; a longer-lasting application of the laser light will not increase the depth of tissue penetration if the power is insufficient. This is why a class-4 laser provides better treatment outcomes than lower-powered lasers, in my opinion. A low-level laser would still produce cellular changes, but it is limited in its depth of penetration. The higher the power, the broader the area and faster the treatment. Technically, you can also hit deeper tissues with the higher-powered laser. The farther down into the tissue the light travels, the more power it has behind it. Another advantage of a high-powered laser comes when treating musculoskeletal type injuries. It's not always easy to find the exact or precise area of the problem that is generating the pain, but the class-4, 15-watt laser can treat a broader area, which ensures the healing energy of the laser hits all possible problem areas. Clinicians can achieve some great results because they don't need to find the precise problem area. The laser itself is small; the entire unit could easily fit in a traveling case, and it weighs about 14 pounds. **Optimal dosage is the single most important parameter for a successful outcome in laser therapy.** Too much or too little energy produces no effect and the matter of correct dosage is very complicated. For this reason it is important for patients to seek out a doctor who is experienced in using lasers because it takes time to find the "optimum window" of treatment dosage. Several things need to be taken into account, such as laser wavelength, power density, type and condition of tissue, whether the problem is acute or chronic, skin pigmentation, and depth of target tissue. The primary factors in laser therapy that determine dosage are power and time. While power is the amount of energy measured at the source of the beam, dosage is the amount of energy delivered to the skin and target tissue. Current industry standards require 4–10 J/cm2 for arthritis conditions. In other words, 4 to 10 joules of energy must be delivered over a cm2, roughly the size of a playing card. In CW mode at 15 watts of power, my laser will put out 900 J of energy in one minute. Spreading this energy over an area roughly the size of a standard playing card would deliver appropriate levels of energy into the body (~10 J/cm2). For example, when treating a large area such as the low back, 6–10 minutes would be the optimum treatment time depending on the size of the patient.

For six years, I have been suffering from arthritis in my left knee due to a fall. Two years ago I began to have sciatic pain and numbness in both of my legs because of the spinal stenosis and another accidental fall. I have tried a lot of other types of treatments (physical therapy and shots) and they were helpful for only a short period of time.

I decided to try the class-4, deep-tissue laser treatments and I am very satisfied with the results. I can now stand up straight and walk a longer distance. Getting up in the morning is easier as I don't have to bend forward to walk because of the numbness. I am 75 percent better and I do not take any more pain pills. The treatments were painless. Thank you, Dr. Alosa, and your staff, Liz Natasha and Amanda. They are very polite, friendly, and efficient.

—Gladys Tom, age 77

A larger patient will have a treatment time closer to 10 minutes and a small patient will have a time closer to 6 minutes, but most patients will be somewhere in between 6-10 minutes. What is very important for patients to understand is that too much treatment time (dosage) will equal no results. There is an optimal therapeutic window of dosage that must be found for each individual patient for maximum results.

WAVELENGTHS AND THE INFRARED ADVANTAGE

As I mentioned earlier, wavelength is another criterion for classifying lasers. The different wavelengths of light and color in the light spectrum are measured. For instance, the red end of the spectrum is 600 nanometers and the near-infrared end of the spectrum is 1100 nanometers. Ideally, you want to find the optimum therapeutic window when treating musculoskeletal problems such as arthritis, which means using the right wavelength. Certain wavelengths penetrate more deeply into the body than others.

The laser I use is an infrared laser, with a dual diode wavelength of 808 nanometers and 980 nanometers. This allows the greatest penetration of photons (which are the mechanism of action for the laser). If the photons can't hit the target tissues in the body, you're not going to get any results. So it's very important to make sure you have the proper wavelength to allow proper penetration of the photons to stimulate the healing process Just as with any other type of light, or rays of light, the photons don't travel in straight lines. Once they hit tissue, there is some refraction to take into account. some photons will be absorbed, and some will scatter or bounce around a little bit. Even if you have the proper wavelength, some photons will scatter, but still enough of them will penetrate the target tissues. Some photons will be lost in the process no matter which wavelength is used. And because they can scatter and bounce around a little bit everyone using a laser, the technician and also the patient, should wear protective eyewear.

THE CELLULAR CHANGES (PHOTOBIOSTIMULATION)

Researchers and scientists have been trying to pinpoint exactly how the laser causes cellular changes, but they're still not 100 percent sure. What they can say with reasonable certainty is that the lasers emit photons and these photons travel into the body and are absorbed by the mitochondria in every cell. This initiates a cascade of events that will reduce pain, reduce inflammation, and increase blood flow. Once the photons are absorbed by the mitochondria, the release of nitric oxide is increased. Nitric oxide is a powerful vasodilator that causes the blood vessels to expand, which enhances oxygenation. The way Viagra works—by releasing nitric oxide—is very similar to the way the laser causes vasodilation and increases oxygenation and blood flow. Photonic energy stimulates the photoreceptor on the mitochondria to increase the reaction time for cytochrome C to become cytochrome C oxidase. This increases the cellular respiration rate, causes a release of nitric oxide, and incites adenosine triphosphate (ATP) production. The term used to describe how the laser causes cellular changes is known as photobiostimulation. I know, I know—another word you have never heard of, but if we break it down into three parts, it becomes very clear what it means. *Photo* means "light" or "photons," and *bio* means "life," so the photons emitted from the laser stimulate cellular repair and cellular regeneration of life. This is one of the major differences between laser therapy and drug therapy. Prescription or over-the-counter drugs do not in any way stimulate the body to heal; they only provide temporary relief, but that relief only lasts as long as you are taking the drug. You will have to keep taking the drug every day for the rest of your life. Because the laser stimulates healing, the pain relief patients experience is long-term, and many of my patients do not need to come back for continued treatment to experience extended pain relief. Let's examine the specifics of how the laser reduces pain.

PAIN REDUCTION PROCESS

There are eight different individual processes that occur with pain reduction. The laser doesn't do just one thing; it does many different things, which makes it very complex. When patients ask me, "So how does the laser work?" they don't understand what a loaded question that is. It is a three-hour course just to learn the principles behind laser therapy. I'll try to give you the shorter version here. First, the laser increases the release of beta-endorphins in the body. These are endogenous peptides that are very powerful, feel-good opioids; the more endorphins in your bloodstream, the better you are going to feel. The "runners' high"—the euphoric feeling runners get after they finish their run—is due to the release of these beta-endorphins. The laser stimulates the release of these feel-good hormones both locally and systemically, all without having to lift a finger or run a mile.

Any kind of pain is decreased when endorphins run through the bloodstream. In fact, the beta-endorphins your body releases from the pituitary gland are more powerful at relieving pain than morphine! The laser not only increases the release of beta-endorphins and nitric oxide but also reduces bradykinin levels. Bradykinins are prevalent in injured tissues and they stimulate nociceptive afferents, which are pain receptors. The higher the bradykinin levels, the more pain. A reduction in bradykinin levels means a reduction of pain.

The laser also normalizes the calcium-potassium ion channels, which have been proven to reduce pain levels. Blocked depolarization of C-fiber afferent nerves is another way laser therapy can reduce pain. C-fiber afferent nerves are one of the many different types of nerves in the body. Yet another important thing the laser can do for pain relief is increase nerve-cell action potential. Everyone still with me? I know I'm using words many readers will not recognize, but since everyone seems to be curious how the laser works, these descriptions are necessary. You can now see the difficulty of answering the question of how the laser works, but once this book is published, I can refer patients to this chapter. This is also a chapter that patients could ask their medical doctor to read. Then, maybe, they will be more apt to recommend class-4 laser therapy to their patients. The following aspects of laser therapy are important for neuropathies or neurogenic pain (nerve caused). Injury or trauma such as OA can impair the resting potential of nerve cells. Normally, the resting potential of nerve cells is ~70 mV (micro volts) but when there is injury or trauma to a joint, that threshold is lowered, meaning the nerve will fire and cause pain from a stimulus that would not normally cause the nerve cells to fire. In other words, nerve cells that would not normally be activated are activated due to the lower threshold caused by the injury. The laser can increase this threshold closer to the normal level of ~70 mV which will help reduce pain levels. Several studies have also shown lasers to be effective in nerve repair through nerve cell regeneration and axonal sprouting. If you read all the testimonials in this book, you will notice lots of patients have had their numbness and neuropathies improved by my treatment program. So the laser does more than reduce pain; it is also useful for patients with diabetic neuropathies or arthritic neuropathies.

REDUCING INFLAMMATION

The class-4 laser does a lot more than just reduce pain. It is also a powerful anti-inflammatory, but it doesn't do just one thing to reduce inflammation. Let me list all of the different proven functions the laser performs to dramatically lower inflammation and edema. The class-4 laser inhibits the synthesis and secretion of inflammatory prostaglandins yet stimulates prostaglandins that have vasodilatory and anti-inflammatory actions. Vasodilation, which we discussed earlier, helps reduce inflammation, but it also reduces interleukin-1, which is a cytokine protein and mediator of the inflammatory response. When the laser reduces this inflammatory mediator, it automatically reduces inflammation at the site of injury because the inflammatory response is limited to the amount of interleukin-1 present. Stabilization of the cellular membrane: CA++, NA+ and K+ concentrations are all positively influenced, partly because of the production of beneficial reactive oxygen species (ROS), which help improve CA++ uptake in the mitochondria. ATP production and synthesis are significantly enhanced, thus influencing cellular repair, reproduction, and functional ability.

The laser also increases leukocytic activity, which is the activity of white blood cells. This results in enhanced removal of nonviable cellular and tissue components, allowing a faster repair and regeneration process. Angiogenesis is important for reducing inflammation

After treatment I am pain-free and have my life back again. I can walk, swim, shop, and look forward to playing with my grandchildren. I experienced low back pain for several years. I had a spinal fusion and still had pain. I also had several physical therapy treatments and still had pain. After laser treatment, I am 90 percent pain-free and feel better every day.

—Julie Cashman, age 69

and for treating failed back surgery syndrome, or any surgery, because of the formation of scar tissue. Angiogenesis is the process of creating new blood vessels in the tissue. Multiple back surgeries can create lots of scar tissue, which can be a primary pain generator. The laser can actually remold that scar tissue into healthy tissue through the process of angiogenesis. This is very helpful to postsurgical patients because there's really nothing else that can help them at that point; they've already had the surgery and the surgery is permanent. The surgeon can't go in and remove it. Conversion of scar tissue to healthy tissue is unique to class-4 laser therapy. I know of no other treatment that has the ability to do that. Many of my patients who suffered from failed back surgery syndrome derive substantial relief from their post-surgical pain through my laser program.

PROMOTES WOUND HEALING AND TISSUE REPAIR

The increased production and synthesis of ATP is helpful in reducing inflammation and it also increases healing by stimulating cells to take up nutrients and get rid of waste by-products faster. It also can increase the rate of cellular mitosis and collagen synthesis. It doesn't stop there; it also activates fibroblasts, chondrocytes, osteocytes, and other tissue repair cells. Chondrocytes are the cells that make up cartilage and arthritis is a disease of the cartilage. I don't think I need to elaborate on how important the laser's ability to stimulate these cells becomes when treating arthritis, but it's not only the cartilage that is stimulated to repair itself. The tendons, ligaments, muscles, and bones are also stimulated. Peripheral nerves are also regenerated, which is helpful for patients suffering from peripheral neuropathies as well as wound healing. The laser enhances leukocyte infiltration.

Leukocytes, or white blood cells, are the part of the immune system; they go in and clean up all the bad stuff such as bacteria and virii. The laser will increase this type of activity as well as macrophage activity. The laser increases neovascularization, which is new blood vessel growth, as well. This encourages fibroblast proliferation, which helps build new tissue. These are all the different things that the laser can do, which is quite remarkable when you think about it. This one little laser can enhance or instigate all these different activities on a cellular level. The reduction of pain and inflammation in addition to the stimulation of tissue healing makes class-4 laser therapy superior to any other type of treatment and is the reason why I am able to get patients with severe chronic arthritis pain better when no one else could.

LASER APPLICATION

This is an important section of the book because I often have patients ask me to do their laser treatments. I will tell you the reader, exactly what I tell patients who ask me to do their treatments.

First of all, If I thought that a doctor must do patient treatments for best results than that's exactly what I would do because getting my patients better is my number one priority, period!

While I was researching this book I found zero research indicating that a doctor must perform treatments for best results. There is only one thing that matters in patient outcomes and that one thing is DOSAGE. The dosage is always the same no matter who does the treatment.

The act of performing a laser treatment on a patient is to be done in a slow "erasure" type movement. If using a handpiece, the handpiece should be held perpendicular to the skin surface about

1-2 inches from the skin and move at a rate of 1-3 inches/second covering the entire circumference of the joint being treated. Treating a patient with a laser is a lot like painting. You are using the red light from the laser to "paint" a body part and that is as simple as it sounds. I'm sure everyone reading this would agree with me that a doctors education and experience is not needed to "paint" a body part. Any employee can be properly trained to be a laser technician but in my office I like to use licensed massage therapists. I prefer them because they are proficient in human anatomy and are already trained and familiar with treating patients.

The handpiece is always in motion and patients should feel a soothing warm sensation during treatment. The patient should notify the technician if they ever feel any thermal discomfort of any kind. If a patient does complain of any discomfort during a treatment, it is easily rectified by moving the wand at a faster rate, or simply lowering the power.

One of the reasons patients ask me to do their treatments is because they say that they felt more heat when I treated them compared to one of my staff. Again this is important because I hear it often from patients, not a lot but it happens enough were I want to address it here. The heat or warmth a patient feels during a treatment is due to the rate of speed the handpiece is moved and the distance it is held from the skin. The slower the handpiece moves and the closer it is to the skin, the patient will feel more heat and vice versa: the faster the handpiece moves and the greater the distance it is held from the skin the patient will feel less heat. What is important for patients to understand is that laser treatments are a photochemical response not a photothermal response. In other words, the heat patients feel during treatment has no connection to patient outcome. It is the photons in the light that stimulates cellular changes and healing. Again, the only thing that matters in patient outcomes is dosage and the dosage is the same no matter how fast or slow the handpiece moves.

If you're a patient, I would recommend going to a doctor that has a qualified staff that treats patients. In my experience, doctors that treat their own patients with a class IV laser don't have enough patients to hire a staff. Not having enough patients equals inexperience. In order for a patient to achieve maximum results the doctor needs to be proficient in accurately diagnosing a patient and equally proficient in setting the optimal dosage.

Many years ago I surgically replaced my left knee. The surgery was successful but shortly thereafter my right knee started giving me trouble as well. I'm an active 83-year-old male who loves to travel and go "holo-holo"; the constant pain was restricting my freedom, my moods, and my quality of life in general. I considered another knee replacement surgery, but due to other medical issues, I was told it would be too risky.

I endured pain and limited mobility for 15 years and then I saw Dr. Alosa's advertisement. I took a chance and started the laser treatment. It was the best decision I ever made!

Today I am virtually pain-free without surgery! I'm not the type of person to write testimonials, but I've made this exception because I'm so thankful to be pain-free again. I hope my words help to convince a few of you to see Dr. Alosa and consider the laser treatment. You may not need to live with pain forever and I hope your results give you the relief that I have found through Dr. Alosa and his exceptional staff!

—**Herbert T. Uyeno, age 83**

STAYING SAFE: WHAT NOT TO DO WITH LASERS

Even though the laser is very safe (I actually know doctors who've taken the class-4 laser and shined it right into their eyes with no protective eyewear just to prove the point that they're not harmful to the eyes), I still advise certain precautions.

- You don't want to treat the lumbosacral area of a pregnant female.
- Avoid epiphyseal lines in children because it may affect the growth plates of children.
- Avoid the testicles.
- Avoid any kind of hemorrhage or cancerous tumor.
- Don't shine the laser directly into the eyes.

Other than these things, the class-4 laser is totally safe to use.

LASERS: THE WAVE OF THE FUTURE

When you consider what the laser has already done in terms of transforming eye care and surgical procedures, and its potential in treating arthritis and other conditions, you'll see that laser therapy really is the wave of the future. I see it every day and the technology involved in creating effective lasers just keeps getting better and better every day. If this all seems too complicated to you, if you found this discussion of wavelengths and cells and infrared spectrum bewildering, here's all you need to know:

- Laser technology is real.
- Laser therapy is safe.
- Laser therapy works.

If you want research, there are over 2500 studies published in journals to back it up. Laser therapy is scientific. It is not snake oil or some fake cure with no science behind it

And, compared to other types of arthritis treatments, which have a lot of serious side effects, laser therapy has none. So not only is it very powerful and effective, but it's very safe. So when patients undergo this type of treatment, they can be 100 percent sure they're not going to come out any worse than when they went in. You can't say that with other types of treatment, especially medically based treatments. As a doctor, I can think of no greater shame than to have a patient get worse from my treatment. I can promise that not one of my patients has ever or will ever have his or her condition worsen with my treatments.

And I believe that's very important for patients, who obviously want to get better; they certainly don't want to get worse. As long as they know that they're not going to get any worse

> I suffered with pain to my lower back for years. I got nerve blocks, massages, acupuncture treatments for a temporary fix. But after receiving laser treatments, I've noticed a big change. No pain—I'm pain-free.
>
> I also have a torn cartilage in two places to my left knee. I was told to have surgery to correct this. But I've been putting it off for more than two years. After receiving laser treatments, my knee seems much better. I don't walk with a limp. I can walk normally and I'm pain free.
>
> After laser treatments I have more circulation and I have more energy. I can do things that I couldn't do before. I love my plants and garden. Now, I'm able to do more and enjoy it. I'm also enjoying my five-year-old grandson and I'm trying to keep up with him. I would recommend this to others because it truly works and no side effects to make it hurt.
>
> **—Jacqueline Young Ganal, age 69**

from this type of treatment, no matter what, they have a little peace of mind. There are some patients that may experience a temporary increase in their symptoms during their treatment process but this is not their condition getting worse, this is their body undergoing a healing process. For some patients the process of cellular repair will temporarily create pain but this is a positive sign that the laser is creating a healing response in the body and that is exactly what we want. I can say with 100% certainty that any temporary increase in a patients symptoms is the result of a patient healing and not their condition worsening. Lasers have been in use for decades and there have been no record of any patient being harmed by a laser. In addition, the best feature of all is that the success rate with laser therapy is very high. In my office, 80 percent of the patients who go through the program get better. Obviously, there's nothing out there that can cure with a 100 percent success rate. Healing is just too complex and each patient is too different for one type of therapy to work effectively on everybody. In fact, I would be very wary of anyone who said that their treatment program got 100 percent of their patients better every single time. So laser therapy doesn't get everybody better, but it gets *most patients* better, which is hard to say for other types of treatments. This is especially true when it comes to producing long-term pain relief for chronic arthritis and not something that's just temporary.

ADDRESSING THE SKEPTICS

In dealing with something that is new to the market, patients are often skeptical. This is especially true for patients who have been to many other doctors and are still in pain. What I tell patients is that they cannot compare class-4 laser therapy to any other treatment they have had because it is the only modality that stimulates the body to heal and therefore cannot be compared to any other treatment. It's not only skeptical patients I encounter but also doctors. Some of my patients go to their doctors to check with them first or get their permission to use the laser. I've had some doctors call me, wanting to see research on the laser's effectiveness. They want to see proper research done on the therapy. But it's not that cut-and-dried. The problem with MDs wanting to see proper research done on laser therapy or any other treatment that is not a drug is that laser manufacturers cannot patent their laser equipment. Since drug companies are allowed to patent their drugs, they can spend the millions of dollars it takes to do a proper scientific study and once the study is published, no other drug company can sell the drug. They basically have a monopoly and can sell the drug for whatever amount they want with zero competition. A laser manufacturer cannot do that. If a laser manufacturer spent the millions it takes to do a study, as soon as the study was published, all of their competitors could use that research to sell their own lasers. This is the reason why laser therapy and other alternative treatments are not researched to the degree that drugs are. MDs don't seem to understand that simple fact and continue to this day to discredit any form of treatment that isn't supported by scientific proof of its effectiveness. If drug companies weren't allowed to unfairly patent their drugs, you would see zero research at drug companies.

I'm all for evidence-based treatments, but when a company pays for its own research, the problem of conflict of interest arises. Anyone familiar with how scientific research is conducted knows a large amount of fraudulent activity is involved in the process. Positive results are often manipulated, making it very difficult to believe them. Moreover, some drug companies research natural supplements, such as vitamin E, with the sole intent of discrediting them. In fact, I just read in the paper today about a research study that claims omega-3 fish oil provides no benefit in preventing heart disease. I have a stack of research papers in my office providing proof—beyond any doubt—that omega 3 fish oil is effective in lowering your risk for heart disease. This is just another attempt by drug companies to devalue their competition. If scientific research were done correctly without fraud and conflicts of interest, it would be a very valuable tool in today's system of health care. Unfortunately, the scientific community is rife with immoral acts and because of that, you cannot believe what any research article states without knowing who paid for the study and the details of how the study was carried out. Because of the aforementioned limitations and outright fraud in today's scientific community, research is not able to provide the skeptics much help with their skepticism. For the skeptics out there, there is only one way to get over skepticism: you must experience the power of 15 watt class-4 laser for yourself. There is no better way to become a believer in laser therapy than to have the laser ease your pain, sometimes in as little as one treatment. There is nothing more powerful than to have patients with chronic arthritis pain feel better after only one treatment. Do you think those patients are going to want to see research after they consulted multiple doctors

> Let me start by saying I was kind of skeptical of laser treatment when my wife brought it to my attention. But I actually started feeling improvement after my second treatment and now I feel almost no pain in my lower back and I'm doing things I haven't done in years thanks to my wife for bringing me here, and the doctor for fixing me. Being able to wake up in the morning with no pain is priceless.
>
> **—James Peck, age 40**

and were still in pain and then received one laser treatment and felt better? Of course not! I see my laser produce "miracles" every day in my office; I do not need to see any research on its effectiveness because I see the effectiveness over and over again.

As a patient, please don't go and ask your doctor if you should try my laser therapy program. Conventional health-care physicians are specialists; they specialize in giving drugs to patients. So if you want to know about a certain drug or a drug's side effect, then of course go get your doctor's opinion, but asking about a treatment your doctor does not provide makes no sense. Doctors don't use this particular laser, so they're not going to spend any of their time researching it. Medical doctors, as I mentioned earlier, get most of their information or knowledge from drug company salesmen or continuing education classes put on by drug companies. So obviously, their information is very biased because these companies are just trying to sell them drugs. Medical doctors don't have the time or the motivation to find the proper evidence that these lasers are effective and scientifically sound and safe. It's very

For many years, I had a severe pain in my neck from an auto accident in my childhood and in my forties, I also started to feel pain in my back (sciatica) but after I received some of the laser treatments, I don't feel that pain like I used to and my back is much better now. I feel light all over my body too. It's amazing how fast the laser treatment works to relieve my pain! After the laser treatment, I can get a good night's sleep, so I feel energetic in the morning, I feel warm inside of my body all night long. Laser treatments are fast and effective, so it saves lots of time in my busy life because it only takes 20 minutes for each treatment. Now, I don't have to get a massage every week and get acupuncture twice a month (at least 1 hour for each treatment).

—Janet Mayerle, age 55

difficult for doctors to obtain unbiased information on treatment that they don't offer in their practice. So when patients ask their doctor to discuss this type of therapy, they can't expect to get an educated response. At the same time, the doctor may feel a little threatened. Just consider this: this patient has been coming to him or her for years with a problem and the patient is still in pain. So that patient leaves to seek care somewhere else. I think doctors would feel threatened by the fact that their patients are leaving them to get treatment somewhere else. Doctors are not that eager to recommend alternative types of therapy, such as laser treatment, because they are afraid they're going to lose their patient and possibly be ashamed that another doctor was able to make their patient better. So I try to tell my patients that there's no need for them to get permission from their doctor to seek care in my office. If they want to know about lasers, they just have to ask me. I'm the expert. The conventional health-care doctors are not experts on laser therapy, and I'm sure they have never authored a book on the subject. I'm hoping this book will help with this problem by giving you another way to get all your questions answered. In the next chapter, I'll take you directly into the treatment room so you'll know exactly what to expect.

Chapter 4

YOUR LASER TREATMENT PROGRAM

A SIMPLE GUIDE

Preparing to experience a new form of therapy can make any patient uneasy when he or she doesn't know what to expect. That especially goes for a therapy such as laser treatment which, due to its newness, can seem like a big question mark to a first-time patient. I have given you a thorough understanding of how a laser works and why laser therapy is so beneficial in the treatment of arthritis. Now let's look at the actual laser treatment process so you'll know what to expect from the moment you walk through the office door. First, you will be greeted warmly by my staff and they will instruct you to fill out our one-page patient intake form. I value my time as much as my patients' time, so I try to keep the duration of the entire new patient process less than 60 minutes. Oftentimes a new patient will be in and out of my office within 45 minutes. We also have a no-wait policy; new patients will be seen within minutes of their appointment time.

YOUR FIRST VISIT

As with any visit to a new doctor's office, your process will begin with my taking your detailed medical history. This line of inquiry, the history, is really the bread and butter of getting to an accurate diagnosis. With a good detailed history, I can come to a proper diagnosis 80 percent of the time. Expect us to spend 10–15 minutes on this part of your visit. I will want to know:

1. How long you have had your problem.
2. What other treatments you have had in the past, with what kind of results.
3. What actions exacerbate your condition, such as sitting, standing, walking, or getting up from a seated position.

Knowing your history will also help me to understand any related conditions you may have. Many such conditions have certain symptoms that go along with them: patients with spinal stenosis, for instance, will have symptoms in both legs, but it would not be pain per se that they feel. Some will have pain, but others will have more like a tight, heavy cramping in their legs. That symptom is very pronounced in stenosis and rules out other conditions.

> I started taking laser treatments and I must say that they have improved my knee 60–70 percent. I used to run marathons but because of arthritis, now I am only walking in my training. But I have seen a big improvement in my golf game. My knee barely hurts after walking and playing golf and this is a big relief to me! I can walk 18 holes of golf and finish without any knee pain. The pain I do feel is soon gone! I would strongly recommend laser treatment to anyone considering it.
>
> **—Brian Moore, age 72**

In terms of movement, certain actions, with back pain or arthritis of the spine, will exacerbate the condition more than others. If you have a disk problem in the lower back, sitting is usually more of a problem than any other position. When you sit, you're increasing the intradiscal pressure and that usually exacerbates disk problems in the lower back. With arthritis in the hip as well as the lower back, walking is usually a problem. Especially with hip arthritis, some patients will walk with a limp. Often I will be able to make a diagnosis after developing a complete and detailed history, including observation, and without carrying out any other type of test, I will take X-rays of patients when necessary.

> With the laser treatments on my knee, I was able to avoid having arthroscopic surgery for a torn meniscus. I was able to continue bowling every week and avoid the six-week recovery period for arthroscopic surgery. Although my knees are not completely pain-free (due to muscle/nerve/spinal pain on my upper calves and behind the knee) after sitting for long periods of time, I feel the meniscus tear has healed. I am able to walk for longer periods of time at the shopping malls and on trips.
>
> —Charlene Yamasaki, age 59

THE EMG TEST

For a patient with any kind of suspected arthritis in the spine, I will do an EMG test. The EMG is unique. A lot of doctors don't incorporate it in their analysis, but it is a good, objective test. EMG stands for electromyography. It is a test that involves placing sensors down the length of and on each side of the spine and using the sensors to read electrical activity (in microvolts) from the muscles. The patient, gowned, sits upright on a stool. The back needs to be bare for the placement of the electrodes (sensors) on the skin. It's totally painless; the patient doesn't feel anything. The sensors are simply reading the electrical activity of the muscles as I place them. In a normal person the reading should be equal on either side of the spine, but if there's a problem with the spine, the two readings on either side of the spine will be different, not symmetrical. Here's why: the nerves that transmit the electrical activity control the muscles. If those muscles or nerves are being affected by arthritis, the condition will change the muscles' response and the generation of electrical impulses. If we have any imbalance on either side of the spine, it will show up in the reading indicated on the EMG printout. The severity of the spinal imbalance and where on the spine it exists will show up on the printout as a colored bar graph indicating the following:

- White=normal
- green=mild problem
- blue=moderate problem
- red=severe problem

This information is particularly helpful if the patient is experiencing symptoms in the extremities. For instance if you have a pain or numbness radiating down into the arm or hand, I can place the EMG sensors over your cervical spine. If we get red colors in the test result, we know there's a severe problem, an indication that your arm/hand problem is actually originating in the cervical spine; the

> I've had this back pain for many years. I had surgery done but the pain didn't go away. Now, with the laser treatment, the pain is substantially less. Now I can do more yard work that I enjoy, without having to suffer the pain each time. I think the pain is 70–80 percent better thanks to the laser treatments.
>
> —**Charles Matsuda, age 70**

problem isn't in your hand or your arm where you are feeling the sensations.

This is important for patients to understand because they often have a hard time comprehending why, if they have arm pain, I am treating their neck, or why, if they have leg pain, I am treating their lower back. All the nerves exiting the spine travel down the arms and legs. So most of the time, probably 90 percent or more, symptoms that radiate into the extremities come from the spine, whether it is at the level of the neck (the cervical spine) or the lower back (the lumbar spine). Using EMG helps me diagnose the exact location of the problem.

One side note: An EMG reading is helpful when dealing with issues such as carpal tunnel syndrome. The majority of numbness or pain in the hands usually comes from the cervical spine, not the wrist. That is one of the reasons why carpal tunnel surgery doesn't have a very good success rate: 90 percent of the time the problem isn't in the wrist. It's actually in the cervical spine. So cutting the flexor retinaculum, which is a tough fibrous band covering the tunnel where the nerves go into the hand, doesn't alleviate the symptoms because the problem wasn't there in the first place.

> I was having pain and numbness from carpal tunnel syndrome on my right hand. After treatment was started, I feel 75 percent better with no pain and minimal numbness. I'm glad that the laser treatment is working and I can cancel the surgery that I was going to have. I sleep much better and I'm able to do more around the house.
>
> **—Donald Tominaga**

THE JOINT EXAM

If the patient's problem is in a particular joint or set of joints instead of the spine, I will examine the joint or joints. Take the knee, for example: I will palpate the joint, or the area of complaint, to check for any tenderness or swelling. This means I am using my hands to press on the joint to locate areas of tenderness, pain, or swelling. I may also do some range of motion tests to give me an idea of the extent of the arthritis. If I suspect arthritis in the neck, for instance, I can put the patient through some range of motion exercises. I have the patient do flexion, which is bringing the head down as far as possible, and then extension, lifting the chin up as far as possible. Then I have the patient rotate his or her head to the right and left, and tilt it to the right and left. If the range of motion is greatly reduced, arthritis is present, probably in the later stages. The advanced stages of arthritis are very easy to see in the hands or in the knees. You cannot see arthritis in the spine without X-rays, but in the knees or the hands you can see if the joint is enlarged, swollen, and deformed. There's no need for an X-ray in such situations; the diagnosis is evident. However, I will use an X-ray for patients who have pain in the hip region or groin

After experiencing arthritis pain for the first time on New Year's Day, I went to the doctor and she had me go to physical therapy. Then I saw Dr. Alosa's ad. I'm glad I tried his laser treatment and have had improved movement in my right knee and am able to straighten my knee and walk without much pain. I have gone back to golf because the swelling around my knee has gone down and I am starting to regain my strength. With little support I can lift myself from a squatting position. I go to the gym and still do my physical therapy. Thank you, Dr. Alosa. You've given me my life back and I hope to enjoy my retirement more.

—Clarence Shibuya, age 69

area. Such pain can be caused by one of two things: a lumbar spine problem causing pain to radiate down into the hip or groin area, or arthritis in the actual hip joints. An X-ray of a patient's hip joints and lower back will provide the information needed to diagnose the exact problem. I have had patients on occasion ask if I need to take an X-ray in order to know if the laser will work for them because they were told they were "bone on bone." Because I have observed this laser work on the most severe and chronic types of arthritis, I know there is no case too severe for laser to work on. I have seen my laser program provide relief for all kinds of "bone-on-bone" patients. For the most part, the only instance where I will X-ray a patient is when I need to diagnose either hip or lumbar spine arthritis.

USING THE LASER

Once I have completed tests and I am confident that the patient has arthritis in a certain area of the body, we move on to using the actual laser on the patient. If the problem is in the lower back, for example, I have the patient lie face down on the treatment table. The patient can be fully clothed, but we will need to pull a shirt/blouse up over the thoracic area and lower pants a couple of inches to expose the lumbar area of the spine.

The laser itself has two different tools we can use, depending on the treatment. The regular hand piece, or wand, is held just an inch or so above the skin. You hold it much as if you were holding a paint brush or marker or eraser. The motion is similar, moving from side to side, typically one to three inches per second. The laser wand is always in motion.

The other tool we use is a massage ball. Just as it sounds, it's a massage ball with a laser in it. You apply the massage ball right on the surface of the skin. Typically, you want to use the massage ball on a trigger point or on acupressure points. The massage ball is good on shoulder problems as well because it's able to move the tissue around so you can get the laser into the deeper structures in the shoulder joint.

During the laser treatment the patient will feel no pain, just the soothing, warm sensation of the laser. Patients are skeptical enough when it comes to lasers, and if they can't feel anything happening during the treatment, that just adds to their skepticism.

Quite often, if we're using the laser on the lower back, patients feel a sensation travel down their legs into their feet. That's a sign that the laser is stimulating the sciatic nerve, which I think is a big help for patients as far as the skepticism goes: feeling something like that happening while they're on the table can only be reassuring to them.

> I have been suffering with knee pain on both my knee caps. I used to have my husband rub my knees so the pain would go away but the pain was still there. I was introduced to deep-tissue laser treatment. I have been treated twice a week for my pain; then I noticed my pain got less and less. Today, both my knees are pain-free. Thank you, Dr. Alosa and staff!
>
> —Emma Ernestburg, Laie, HI

The length of a single laser treatment depends on the area of the body being treated. For instance, a wrist is not going to take as much time as a hip. A hip is going to take 10 to 15 minutes to treat; a wrist will take 5 to 6 minutes. When you're done, there are no restrictions on what you can or can't do after the treatment. Just do your normal activities and keep an eye on the area and be wary of how you feel. For example, are there things that you are now able to do that you weren't able to do prior to the treatment? We will schedule you to return for your follow-up typically within two to five days.

THE FOLLOW-UP

Some patients feel relief after the very first treatment. Some patients even feel relief as soon as they get off the table. They say, "Wow, my back feels better already" or "My knee feels better already." I would say probably 40 percent or 50 percent of my patients will feel something immediately after the first treatment, which helps them get over any skepticism they may have had. When a patient obtains relief after the first treatment, that is obviously a good sign, but what is important for patients to understand is that the relief experienced from just one treatment is mainly due to the laser's anti-inflammatory effects and this is usually only a temporary relief, lasting anywhere from a few hours to a week. So the relief patients get from the first treatment is temporary, but the

This laser treatment is the only thing that works so quickly. I wish I'd known about it sooner. I can now walk and do a lot of things without my knee brace. I don't wrap my knee with towels and tape at night to protect It from the cool air. I can sleep pain-free and get some rest. I don't need to buy any more pain pills and cream. I tried anything that said it would stop the pain. I'm now back on the driving range. My golf swing made my knee hurt so bad I had to stop. I will soon be back on the golf course. Bowling without my knee brace helps my game. I'm swimming and not afraid of the cold water making my knees painful. I'm planning a hunting trip for pigs next month. Three months ago at age 61, I thought my life was going to only be dealing with knee pain. But after laser treatment I feel 10 to 15 years younger and feel like I can do anything, and I'm trying to!

—Milton Mento

laser can provide long-term pain relief by stimulating the body to heal. The healing process, however, takes time. Because of this, most patients experience the most progress in the second half of their treatment plan. One or two treatments will not provide lasting results unless the injury is acute. Most of my patients have chronic arthritis. When they return for the follow-up visit, I can evaluate their response to the treatment. I will then use that evaluation to make my recommendation for a treatment program, which includes information on:

- the number of treatments the patient will need
- the duration of the program
- the frequency of the patient's visits to my office
- the cost of the treatment

A TREATMENT PROGRAM

My laser programs cannot have a one-size-fits-all approach. Every patient is different depending on his or her condition and a number of other factors including: patient's age, diagnosis, how long the patient has had the problem,

I have had two knee operations to repair a tear in my knee. I have been living with pain for a long time. After reading Dr. Alosa's laser treatment testimonies in the newspaper, I decided to try it. After my first trial treatment, I did experience some pain relief. I decided to take the treatment plan Dr. Alosa recommended. After the fourth treatment, I was 30 percent pain-free. After the sixteenth treatment I was 90 percent pain-free. It felt GREAT! I did not need to take pain medication and wear a brace. I can stand and walk up steps without pain. I play golf twice a week. I no longer wear a brace or take medication for pain. I am pain-free. I can live a normal life. Thank you very, very much, Dr. Alosa. I'm happy with my life. You made me a new man.

—**Clifford Horita, age 75**

health history, and skin type. Acute problems such as a sprained wrist or tennis elbow will respond to treatment a lot faster than a chronic condition such as degenerative arthritis that a patient has had for years. An acute injury to a small joint such as the wrist or elbow requires about six to eight treatments. But a patient with chronic pain will have a treatment program that is more extensive, usually 10–25 treatments, sometimes over 30. Again, each patient has to be evaluated separately to get an accurate diagnosis and history to determine an individual treatment plan. Chronic conditions, especially those involving a larger part of the body, such as the lower back or the hip, will most likely require the patient to have 12 to 30 treatments. The patient comes in at least three times a week for the first two weeks of a program. If a patient is on a 20-treatment program, for example, he or she will start off with three treatments a week for the first week and then go down to two times a week for the remainder of the program. Laser treatments are cumulative, meaning each treatment builds on the previous one. So the more treatments the patient receives, the more effective the laser becomes and the more progress the patient makes. Because of this build up, we usually see patients make the most progress in the second half of the treatment program. We expect to see the most progress from treatment 10 on because of the therapy's cumulative nature. It's important to understand this because many patients do see some results sooner than they expected. However, and I've seen this with many patients, they will start to feel so much better after five or seven treatments, or whatever it may be, that they want to stop treatments.

I explain why stopping is not a wise decision: the laser provides long-term pain relief by enabling the body to heal itself on the cellular level. The cells are repairing and regenerating, but it is a process that takes time. If the patient stops treatment as soon as he or she starts to feel pain relief, the healing process will be incomplete. Continuing with your treatment program is the only way to ensure that you get long-term pain relief. I have had patients who do not complete their programs and they end up coming back two to six months later because they say the pain is back. I tell them it is because they did not complete my recommended program. The good thing is that because they have already had a series of treatments in the past, they respond faster to the second round and can again feel better quickly. However, it is a lot easier, more effective, and less expensive to just follow through with my original recommendations to ensure the best results and the best long-term outcome. Another issue that is important for patients to understand is that if, for instance, they are on their tenth treatment and have yet to obtain any significant relief, they become discouraged and want to stop treatment. But stopping at this point is a mistake because, as I mentioned earlier, the laser treatments are cumulative—they tend to get more effective the more treatments the patient has. The problem with stopping care is that patients may be stopping just as they are about to break through and start feeling better. What I usually do in these cases is increase the treatment frequency to three times a week,

> Searching for every treatment option available had been a quest for me the past five years. I needed to find the best treatment that would allow me to have the best quality of life. From the very first laser treatment I've noticed a huge different in both knees. I was able to sleep right through the night with no pain. Being hopeful, optimistic, and assertive, I needed to be patient and committed to whatever appointments the doctor gave me and stick to the routine. I now am able to go the distance and take longer walks with no pain.
>
> **—Donna Takahashi-Gomes, age 56**

or have the patient come for treatment three or four days in a row. That is usually enough to get patients over the hump, so to speak, and they usually start to feel better with that increase in the treatment frequency.

BUT DO I HAVE TO KEEP COMING BACK FOREVER?

Many patients ask this question because they think laser therapy is similar to getting a chiropractic adjustment. With chiropractic adjustments, patients have to keep coming back because the benefits of the treatment are lost if regular adjustments are not made. It's like exercise: you get the benefits of exercise when you exercise, but when you don't exercise, you start to lose the benefits. But laser therapy is different. With laser therapy, most of my patients who complete my recommendations don't need to return. It is a good idea, though, to come back on a maintenance basis, perhaps 6–10 treatments a year, just to ensure that your pain stays reduced and you have less chance of the pain coming back, but most patients don't. In fact, I don't require patients to come back except for those who have

> The benefits of laser treatment are many. I can walk without my knee stiffening; it feels free to move. I rarely take any pain medications. I also was saved from having another knee surgery. Having surgery was a very painful process with long months of therapy. With laser therapy, I didn't have to take off from work and it doesn't take long to do the treatments. I am confident in doing my job, which I enjoy. I feel I am more independent. I can do a lot of things on my own. I love traveling, which I know I can do more of in the future. I am happier; it's giving me hope. I participate in sports like fishing and swimming.
>
> **—Darlene Natividad, age 58**

failed back surgery syndrome. These are patients who have had surgery in the past and still have pain. Patients, especially those who have had multiple surgeries, often need continued treatment and will most likely have some degree of chronic back pain for the rest of their life just because of the damage surgery does and the scar tissue formation that results. Fortunately, laser therapy works very well on these types and some of my failed back surgery patients get profoundly better. For these types of patients and for those who suffer from severe degenerative arthritis, I recommend some type of maintenance plan. This is especially important for patients with rheumatoid arthritis because their condition will flare up after periods of remission.

I have been suffering from chronic neck pain the last five years to the point that when sitting in a chair, I would need pillows to support the neck. That was the only way I could get relief from the pain and unfortunately it became a way of life. From the first treatments of laser I started feeling pain reduction. Over a period of six weeks I have been pain-free. Sometimes I have sore muscles in the neck area, but I'm pain-free. It changed my life; my sleeping has improved 100 percent. No more Advil, and I can play golf without neck pain. I have also been able to sit without any neck support.

—David Zuccolotto, age 75

THE BEST OF BOTH WORLDS

But for the most part, after their initial recommendation of care, patients don't need to come back, and they don't come back. It's really the best of both worlds to have a treatment that is safe and effective and you don't need to keep returning for it to work. In fact, lasers have been in use for over 30 years and not one known patient has been harmed or hurt by laser therapy. The safety record of lasers is amazing; you can't say that about a lot of other treatments for arthritis.

When patients ask me if they have to keep coming back, they're definitely stunned when I tell them, for the most part, no. Usually they're surprised because just about every other doctor they go to, they have to keep going back and that's something that turns off patients. They don't want to keep coming into the doctor's office to get treatments. They want it taken care of and taken care of for good. This is what the laser can offer for most conditions, especially the acute and less chronic conditions. But it also works well with patients suffering from severe degenerative chronic arthritis.

The future of laser therapy is very bright. It's just a matter of time before it's used in a lot more doctor's offices. For now it's pretty satisfying for me to be able to work with these people and have such positive outcomes.

My name is Gene Naipo Sr. I am 84 years and of Hawaiian ancestry. When I read Dr. Alosa's laser treatment article I was curious, in hopes it would prolong my life for a few more years. When I scheduled my first appointment I was open minded, excited and yet skeptical at the same time. My first question to Dr. Alosa was, "can the treatment prolong my life two years?" He looked at me with a gentle smile. Once I started my treatment, I soon discovered the answer. It came on two words, RELIEF and HOPE!! Benefits from the laser treatments. Better quality of sleep, better mobility getting in and out of bed, I feel more stable in my daily routines and this laser experience has affected my overall well-being, positively. Mahalo Dr. Alosa

—Gene Naipo, age 84

PAIN AND THE HEALING PROCESS

As we discuss positive outcomes, it's important that you understand exactly what happens in the healing process. Sometimes with laser treatment, patients, especially those with neuropathies (nerve-related problems), can experience an exacerbation of their symptoms. It doesn't happen a lot, but 5–10 percent of patients will experience this and not necessarily with the first treatment. They can be five or six treatments into their program and then all of a sudden their pain feels a lot worse or their condition seems to be a lot worse. The patients are shocked and they think the laser is making them worse. But it's actually a good sign because the laser stimulates a healing response and for some patients, when they go through a healing process, it doesn't feel good. Fortunately, that process is temporary and once they get through that healing process they will feel much better than before. What's happening here is partly what's called retracing.

Both sides of my hip are now pain-free after laser treatments. I'm also having laser treatments on my left ankle (which I fractured about two years ago) as I had some pain in that area and it is now so much better after only five laser treatments. It's so nice to be pain-free when I get up in the mornings. Dr. Alosa is also treating my arthritic fingers and so far they are much better as I use them to play my ukulele once a week. The best thing about the laser treatment is that it is pain-free. It has been 3 ½ weeks and I have not taken any pain pills since I started with the laser treatments. I can now do the things that I dreaded doing like clean the toilets, mop the floors and sweep the outside cement areas as my hips are now pain-free. I can now rub my fingers (both hands together) and there is no pain. I couldn't do that without my pain pills. I wanted to be free of taking any pain pills and I think laser treatments are the answer to my prayers.

—Janet Yokoyama, age 72

Your body will retrace the actual injury, and when it does that, it will cause an exacerbation of the symptoms or an increase in pain. It is not that the condition itself is getting worse; it just means that the body is healing and that doesn't always feel good. However, great pain relief will follow shortly. My patients who experience this always come back and say, "You know what, doc, you were right. Yesterday was the best day I've ever had; it feels much better." So I actually like it when patients tell me their pain is worse because I know they're going to be feeling a lot better soon.

It's important that my patients understand the healing process. It is also important that my patients communicate to me any concerns they have about pain or the treatment so they can be addressed. Some of my patients drop out of care but won't tell me why. When we call them, they just say, "I want to stop care." Those patients I can't help because they didn't finish their recommended treatment program and they never told me what their problem was.

But I do want to help, so please know this: as long as my patients make the commitment to me and follow through with my recommendations, I always will make the same commitment to them. This means I will work with them until I get them better, or until we hit the maximum therapeutic benefit that, with the laser, is probably right around 30–35 treatments but I have had a patient who took over 60 treatments to respond. If I have, for instance, a patient on a 20-treatment program, and we get to the twentieth treatment, but the patient is only 5 percent or 10 percent better, I will keep working with that patient—up to about 30 or more treatments—to see if I can achieve more pain relief for him or her. Sometimes I'll increase the frequency of treatments. If the patient is coming into my office two times a week, I'll have him or her come in three times a week for the next two weeks, and usually that is enough; just about every time, the patient will experience greater pain relief. I usually do those extra treatments at no cost because I like to give more than what patients expect or paid for.

I've been suffering from pain in my knees for more than 10 years. I took all kinds of meds prescribed by my doctor, like glucosamine, etc., to no avail. On my laser treatment program I've felt so much better. My pain is significantly reduced in my both knees. No more walking with a limp! I'm back to almost normal and I'm now pain-free. These laser treatments have relieved my pain tremendously.

—Emosi Finau, age 69

When you come to my office, it is my hope that you'll feel we are on the same team, working toward the same goal: getting you better. I only ask that you stay as focused and committed to your healing as I will be.

Chapter 5

HOME CARE TACTICS: PROTECTING YOUR BODY FROM ARTHRITIS

YOUR BODY: YOU ONLY GET ONE

Recently I read a biography of Warren Buffet, the billionaire investor, and was blown away by his thoughts on caring for the body. He said if you have one car for a lifetime, wouldn't you take really good care of it? You would because you would only have this one car and it has to last you a lifetime. This is exactly the same position we're in with our bodies. We each have just one body and it's got to last us a lifetime. If you don't take care of your body now, it's going to be a wreck 20 years later, just as the car would be. It's what you do today that determines how your body will operate 10–20 years from now. However, it seems to me a lot of patients take better care of their cars than their bodies, and that's a big mistake because you can't replace your body. You can always replace the car, but if you don't do the right things and take care of your body now, you're going to find yourself in some real pain, and you'll have some real health problems down the road.

In this chapter you will learn how to take care of your body when you have arthritis. Obviously, you can't prevent joint damage if joint damage has already been done, but you can protect your body against further damage. What is realistic? What can you do? While there is nothing available on the market that can reverse damage done to a joint, you can learn more about the damage itself, and what causes it, to keep from worsening the condition.

The laser treatments have significantly helped me reduce the pain threshold in my left wrist/hand plus right-hand fingers. Since my rheumatoid arthritis (RA) attack in 2003, plus severe osteoarthritis (OA) in my left wrist until now, I have suffered constant pain and major pain flare-ups in my hands. I was severely physically challenged with doing daily chores or with everything I do with my hands. I couldn't even hold on to a large dinner plate in a dinner buffet line; it was too painful. Now I hardly have pain flare-ups in my left wrist/hand and only experience minor discomfort working with two hands. Now, I no longer need to take extreme medical treatment for my left wrist. I resisted and did not undergo surgery for pain relief as recommended. I do not take any more cortisone painkillers injections for immediate, temporary pain relief. I do not take painkillers anymore—Celebrex, Bextra, Tylenol, codeine, or even a simple OTC Advil. These were my daily routines for pain management and I hated this protocol. The laser treatments have significantly improved my quality of life—to be pain-free. I can go on and do my main hobbies: deep water ocean and shoreline fishing. I can do—and enjoy—shop work with my hand tools again. What a great feeling. Mahalo to Dr. Jerry Alosa and his professional staff for having helped me turn a new chapter in my life style.

—**Ronald Chun, age 74**

INFLAMMATION VS. WEAR AND TEAR

Some exciting new research came out that, for the first time, shows how osteoarthritis is actually the result of an autoimmune attack on the joints, very similar to rheumatism and other autoimmune types of arthritis. This debunks the "wear and tear" theory for osteoarthritis which claimed that OA was always age-related. Researchers from Stanford have shown OA is accompanied by the same pathological, proinflammatory immune factors involved in rheumatoid arthritis. The Stanford team's discovery was first presented in late 2011.

These 25 scientists concluded that the development of OA is in great part driven by low-grade inflammatory processes. Specifically, the researchers discovered that the body launches an orchestrated, powerful attack on the synovial joints by signaling proteins normally used to fight infections. This autoimmune response, they reported, plays a key role in OA onset. So what the Stanford team found is that low-grade inflammation is not merely an early symptom of arthritic cartilage destruction; it is in fact the trigger that causes it!

OA was long thought to be an effect of "wear and tear" on the joints. That's why most medical doctors will tell their patients that they will just have to live with the pain of OA because it is inevitable and there is nothing they can do about it. On the other hand, rheumatoid arthritis is known to be an inflammatory autoimmune disease that arises when the body mistakenly attacks its own tissue, the synovial lining of joints in particular. Now we know that both OA and RA arise from the same proinflammatory immune factors. These researchers found that the body's killer T-cells are attracted to "exposed" collagen within the synovial lining. Normally collagen elicits no immune response, but it is exposed collagen that immune cells mistakenly identify as invasive, foreign molecules. In addition to killer T-cells being activated, inflammatory cytokines are released that actually draw in more killer T-cells. These cells begin to bombard the exposed collagen in the cartilage with toxic chemicals in an effort to destroy it. This process creates oxidative stress and further inflammation in the joints. Over time, your immune system continues these biomolecular attacks on your cartilage. That leads to further damage and destruction.

The researchers found that it is only "exposed" collagen that attracts the killer T-cells. The million-dollar question is why or how is the collagen exposed? Is the collagen exposed naturally? If it is, then why does the immune system wait to attack? Wouldn't it attack early on in life and wouldn't that lead to 5- and 10-year-olds with inflamed joints? My guess is the collagen becomes exposed when the cartilage begins to crack and break down. This leads me to believe that OA still has some sort of "wear and tear" process to it and once the cartilage begins to break down, the process switches to an autoimmune process.

> I have been suffering severe lower back pain for over six years now. I visited different doctors and specialists but no one seemed able to help me. My doctor prescribed a strong pain killer but it did not help me a lot. I bought myself exercise equipment, a detox machine, a biomat, and some heating pads, but all of this did not help. My pain was so severe that walking from my bedroom to the kitchen, I had to use my cane or hold on to the wall to get there. I also visited an acupuncturist and several chiropractors, but again, it seemed nobody could help me. A couple of months ago, I read an article in the paper regarding this certain doctor. I did not wait any longer; I called and made an appointment right away. Thank you, Dr. Alosa. I am feeling much better now. I can walk without my cane or without any assistance. I can also babysit my granddaughter now. I am having some pain from time to time but it does not bother me that much anymore; again, thank you, Dr. Alosa.
>
> **—Erlinda Gonzales, age 72**

So our focus here is to learn what you can do to care for a body already damaged in this process. The ideas in this chapter should help to increase your response to the laser therapy. By doing some of the things we discuss here, you will have better results and a greater opportunity to feel better both during the treatment and afterward. Why? Because taking good care of yourself at home is key to your long-term relief.

TOP FOUR THINGS YOU CAN DO AT HOME

When it comes to dealing with arthritis, in particular osteoarthritis, patients have four basic tactics in their arsenal that they can work on at home:

- weight control
- controlling inflammation
- stretching and exercise

Weight control and inflammation are strongly influenced by the same variable: diet. So let's spend some time here discussing, not dieting, but an optimal way of eating that you can continue throughout your life.

THE CHINA STUDY

The 2004 book *The China Study*, written by T. Collin Campbell, Jacob Gould Schurman Professor Emeritus of Nutritional Biochemistry at Cornell University, and his son, Thomas M. Campbell II, a physician, is a bestseller that describes the largest, most comprehensive nutritional study ever done on humans in history. It studied the effects of diet on people, specially examining the relationship between the consumption of animal products and illnesses such as cancer, diabetes, coronary heart disease, obesity, autoimmune disease, osteoporosis, brain disease, and macular degeneration. The study observed more than 350 variables of health and nutrition with surveys from 6,500 adults in more than 2,500 counties across China and Taiwan, and conclusively demonstrates the link between nutrition and all of the conditions listed above. It also revealed that proper nutrition can have a dramatic effect on reducing and reversing these ailments as well as curbing obesity. The China Study researchers found beyond any kind of doubt that people who ate the most animal protein got the most chronic disease. On the other side of that, people who ate the most plant-based foods or plant-derived protein were the healthiest and tended to avoid chronic disease. I know no one wants to hear that, especially in this American culture where we all love our steak and

> I can now do things at work and at home that I would not do otherwise without great discomfort to my lower back and hips, simple things like walking, tying my shoes, playing with the kids. I couldn't do any of these things without a lot of pain. Then I read about Dr. Alosa's treatment. I had to try it out. Nothing was working—steroids shots, painkillers. They did nothing to help me with coping with the pain every day. After the treatment, I can stand, walk, exercise, run up and down stairs, carry the kids on my back; work has improved 100 percent. I can tie my own shoes now; I go to the beach a lot. The laser treatment is a miracle to me, for I have no pain at all. I am very happy with the results. I wish I knew about this sooner, for the suffering of low back pain for 30 years is gone. God Bless you, Dr. Alosa. You are a godsend. I would recommend this treatment for all the people who suffer from chronic pain.
>
> —Timothy K. Candelaio, age 55

potatoes. But the study showed that animal proteins will increase inflammation, and that inflammation leads not only to weight gain and an increase in arthritic symptoms, but also to hypertension, diabetes, heart disease, and cancer. It's a direct link. In fact a lot of the major chronic degenerative conditions people face in this country are influenced, and can even be reversed, through a vegetarian diet based on plants and limiting the amounts of animal proteins that are consumed.

THE HORMONE FACTOR

Now we know that when you eat animal proteins, inflammation is processed. But how exactly does that happen? There are three groups of hormones called prostaglandins that are responsible for the inflammatory response in humans. You can break or classify them as prostaglandins 1, prostaglandins 2, and prostaglandins 3. Prostaglandins 1 and 3 are good, they are anti-inflammatory. However prostaglandins 2 are the bad ones, so to speak. They are the ones that are proinflammatory, they create more inflammation in the body. Prostaglandin 2 is found in a lot of red meat and dairy products. These products are high in arachidonic acid, the main culprit in setting off a proinflammatory response.

By eliminating these types of proteins from your diet, you can automatically reduce the level of the inflammation in the body. As we have already discussed, inflammation is a major issue of arthritis and just by changing the diet, you can lower inflammation in the body and in turn lower your risk of developing one of the leading causes of death in this country, such as heart disease and cancer.

A side note: the China Study researchers found that cancer is heavily influenced by a diet particularly high in animal protein. The more animal protein someone consumes, the greater the chance they have of (1) developing cancer and (2) of cancer proliferating very rapidly. But you can actually reverse that entire process just by reducing the amount of animal protein that you consume. So a plant-based diet isn't just good for reducing inflammation; it's also quite effective at lowering your risk of the major diseases that afflict just about all Americans as they get older.

THE FRAMINGHAM STUDY

In the 1970s researchers began a very large study in the town of Framingham, Massachusetts. They took a group of people living in this town and studied them extensively for over 30 years. Most people know this study in terms of its findings about the heart. But one of the studies they did in this particular group involved examining what effect patients' weight had on their arthritis symptoms or the chances of their getting arthritis. What they found was the heaviest men had about a 1.5x greater risk of knee arthritis compared to the lightest men. Among women, the findings were actually worse: the heaviest women had more than double the risk of knee arthritis compared to the lightest women.

The researchers also did a follow-up study in the 1990s and those results showed that every 10 pounds of extra weight increases your risk of osteoarthritis by 1.4. So it's clear that excess weight increases your chances of arthritis. This means that just by controlling your weight, you reduce your chances of developing arthritis to a great degree. While weight is obviously something we can control, doing so isn't easy. Exercise, for instance, is important, but if you have an arthritic knee, it probably hurts to do any kind of weight-bearing exercise such as walking or jogging. It is difficult for most patients with advanced cases of arthritis to exercise. But with diet, that's not the case. Anyone can watch what he or she eats and adhere to a healthy, anti-inflammatory diet to help control weight.

THE CARB QUESTION

I don't think there's any one subject that the public is more confused about than diet. Every time you turn around, there's a new diet book out promoting low carbs and then there's another one promoting high carbs and then there's low protein, high protein, low fat, high fat. It goes on and on! So it's very confusing for patients and for the public in general. But the China Study found out that it didn't matter how many carbohydrates you consumed. The consumption of animal protein by far had the most detrimental effects on human health compared to any other factor that they studied. As far as the concerns of the ratio of car-

I am very active woman. I play tennis a lot, hiking, swimming, running, zumba, etc. Unfortunately, I did overdo and injured my left knee, which was diagnosed as a meniscus tear and I also hurt my upper thigh. I had so much pain and couldn't run, bend, or lift my leg, and it was even hard to walk sometimes. Instead of surgery, I tried this laser treatment. First, halfway through, my pain came and went, but after that, I could tell that I was getting better every day. I finished the treatment. Now, I can run like a teenager, bend my knee, climb mountains without any pain. Unbelievable! My life is great if I can stay in very good health—and without doing any exercise, I can't live. Then I got injured ... had to go to surgery ... but after I had a big surgery done some time ago, I did not want to have that again. Then I found out about laser treatment. I had no idea it would work on my leg, but I tried and prayed. Now, after treatment, I can get back to my routine—no more pain, suffering, and frustration. I'm enjoying my life! I feel like I'm a teenager! Thank you!

—Utami Adams, age 61

bohydrates to protein and fat, most of the food you consume should come from plants and fruits. That's the bottom line. If you want to go a step farther, the plants or the vegetables should be eaten raw for the best outcome. Research recommends that 80 percent of the vegetables should be eaten raw or uncooked. I know that would not be very appealing to many people and probably not a diet many would stick with. If you're not in a health crisis, it can be very hard to eat a diet like that. It's not as tasty as a diet that's high in fat and animal proteins. But when faced with a health emergency, whether you have severe degenerative arthritis, or heart disease, or cancer, you may think differently. A good diet is the most powerful weapon you have against disease and sickness. This isn't my opinion or my belief or anyone else's opinion or belief. This is a fact because it has been studied extensively and proven beyond any type of doubt. When you know what the ideal diet is, you don't have to worry about counting calories or what percentage of your food should come from carbo-hydrates or what percentage can come from fat. You simply eat a vegetarian diet with very low or virtually no animal protein. But that doesn't mean you go without protein. You get it from just the plants and the vegetables that you eat. Another misconception is that people think they need protein and they need meat as a source of protein. But the study found that wasn't true. You don't need that much protein to begin with, and you can get plenty of protein from a plant-based diet, especially by consuming beans and lentils. In fact, the protein in a plant-based diet is actually a higher-quality protein than animal protein.

GETTING SPECIFIC: DIET CHOICES

Our discussion so far has been about what you can do in general for a good diet. But there are other choices you can make specifically that will help patients with arthritis. To make these choices you'll have to pay closer attention to the food you pick up in the grocery store. One of the things you'll want to be on the lookout for is partially hydrogenated fats. You don't want to consume or eat them, but they're found in almost any kind of packaged foods such as cookies, cake mixes, flours, and crackers—basically, anything that comes in a can, a box, or a bag. To check for them, you have to read the product label: anything that contains hydrogenated or partially hydrogenated oils and fats—for example, partially hydrogenated soybean oil—don't eat it. Probably the one category that has the most partially hydrogenated fats is spreads and margarines. They are not real butter. Real butter contains the real fats that you find in nature. Our body is built to digest and to assimilate this kind of fat. However, these partially hydrogenated fats are created by boiling the fats at a very high temperature. Hydrogen gas is bubbled through them at very high temperatures, which converts the original cis form of these fats, and they become partially hydrogenated, changing their structure. They actually go from a cis form to a trans form. The transformation causes a problem because trans fats inhibit certain enzymes that are necessary for your body's normal metabolism of fats. They do this for a long time in the body because they are not found in nature; your body has a hard time digesting them and getting rid of them.

This too has been borne out by research. Walter Schmitt, a chiropractor who has studied hydrogenated fats and oils, found that when you eat normal cis fats, the body metabolizes half of them in 18 days. But when you eat trans fats the body requires 51 days to metabolize half of them. This means that half of the trans fats you eat today will still be inhibiting enzymes in your body 51 days from now. So you can picture that as you consume potato chips: your body will be trying to digest the trans fats in those chips 51 days from now!

As these hydrogenated fats continue to hang around in your system, they interfere with the normal breakdown or production of prostaglandins—prostaglandin 1, prostaglandin 2, and the prostaglandin 3, which we talked about earlier. In fact, these fats increase the level of prostaglandin 2s, the "bad" family of prostaglandins. That leads directly to inflammation. Of course, inflammation is one of the main things we want to control when it comes to arthritis and arthritis-type pain. But the trans fats will block the production of prostaglandin 1 and prostaglandin 3. By default, prostaglandin 2 substances are produced unopposed, so this creates a prostaglandins-2 imbalance, which will contribute to the production of chronic disease because just about every chronic disease has been linked to inflammation in the body. The greater the levels of inflammation in the body, the greater the chance of developing a chronic disease. But by not consuming trans fats, you can lower inflammation in the body, and lower your risk of chronic disease.

This information is important to consider if you don't want to totally abandon an animal-protein diet. It's something else you can do in addition to the diet choices we've already talked about because I don't expect everyone to read this book and go out and be a vegetarian. But you can make different choices and limit harmful aspects of your diet. You may not be able to limit all the animal protein in your diet, but you can watch or eliminate trans fats.

STAYING VIGILANT

Just being aware of trans fats is vitally important because most people are probably consuming lots of them without knowing it. If you walk down the aisles in a typical grocery store, just about every shelf is going to be full of foods that are in a package or in a box or in a can, and that is where you find all the trans fats. Unless you're eating a vegetarian diet, you're going to be eating a lot trans fats just because that's a typical American diet. These foods are everywhere including fast food restaurants. A lot of fast foods are loaded with trans fats because they are generated in the frying oils. Just by eliminating those foods, you will see your symptoms relieved or diminished. Be aware of trans fats and avoid them as best you can because they're toxic.

HITTING THE RESET BUTTON

Diet and environment causes 95 percent of disease. That means virtually all disease is caused by lifestyle factors, whether it's the diet you choose to consume or the environment you live or work in. The typical American diet contains a lot of toxins, whether from trans fats or pesticides, herbicides, mercury, and other heavy metals. They end up in our bodies from the food we eat or the water we drink. The most effective way that people can detox their bodies without the help of a doctor is to do a Master Cleanse. If you've consumed a lot of animal protein or prescription drugs, you already have a lot of toxins in your body. When I have patients in this situation, I usually recommend they hit the reset button by doing a fast or a cleanse. This is a regimen, lasting anywhere from 7 to 40 days, during which you abstain from eating any solid food and allow the body to detox and reset. I do them regularly myself, and the fast I have found to be the most effective is known as the Master Cleanse.

THE MASTER CLEANSE

The Master Cleanse was developed in the 1970s by a man named Stanley Burroughs. He wrote about it in a small book outlining the simple process. During the cleanse, you consume no solid food. All of your calories/energy comes from drinking a lemonade mixture made from spring water, freshly squeezed lemon juice, high quality (grade A or B) maple syrup, and cayenne pepper. The cayenne pepper is optional. You also consume a laxative tea in the evenings and mornings to help move toxins out of the body through bowel evacuation. (Some people, instead of drinking the laxative tea in the morning, will do a saltwater flush by drinking a quart of water mixed with two teaspoons of Celtic sea salt, but this is optional.) For more details on how to do the cleanse, you can go to http://themastercleanse.com/.

The Master Cleanse can be done from seven days all the way up to 40 days. Most people do 7–10 days, but either way, this cleanse is probably the single healthiest thing anybody could ever do for himself or herself. I do two seven-day cleanses a year and I can't say enough about the beneficial effects I get from it. Many people don't understand that it is possible to function without solid food. They think if you don't eat any solid food for a week that you'll be sluggish and fatigued. But the truth is the exact opposite! You actually have so much more energy that your body just feels much better. You also think a lot more clearly. I usually get more done in a week when I'm on a Master Cleanse than I probably do in a typical month when I'm not on the cleanse. You have more energy, but you also have so much more time simply because you're not dealing with food. It's surprising to realize how much time you actually spend figuring what to eat, going to the grocery store to get it, making it, and then eating it, and cleaning up after.

In the Chinese culture, it's a lot more common to fast and cleanse and it's done every quarter—four times a year. I think that is a little excessive, but if I have a patient who is 60 years old and has had a bad diet with lots of fast foods and animal protein, it would probably be warranted for that patient to do fasts that often. All these toxins that we eat, breathe in, and consume are trapped inside the tissues of the intestines, colon, and liver – and it's exactly those toxins that will create sickness and disease. The premise behind the Master Cleanse is that your body goes directly into cellular repair mode as soon as the body is not digesting food.

As I mentioned earlier, with this cleanse, you don't eat any solids foods and you also drink a laxative tea, once in the morning and once at night, which helps remove toxins from the body. The tea goes all the way through your intestines and your colon. Just by getting rid of these toxins, your body is going to be a lot healthier and will start to function a lot better. The Master Cleanse is very safe. You can do it for up to 40 days (I actually know a woman who did it the full 40 days). All the vitamins and minerals that your body needs are in the syrup and the lemon juice. Your body doesn't need any more than that. Some people criticize the Master Cleanse because it doesn't have any protein in it but, as we just discussed with the China Study, the amount of protein that we need is minimal. If you're only doing the cleanse for seven days, you may lose a little muscle mass from protein loss, but it's minimal and nothing to be concerned with. You will build it right back up after the cleanse is done. The Master Cleanse is probably the most efficient way to rid the body of toxins because you're not eating any other toxins while you're doing it. With other cleanses, you still eat food, and you take pills to help cleanse the body. But this is nowhere as effective because you're still consuming toxins in your food that your body must try to excrete. That takes up energy that the body could use to get rid of the toxins built up over the years. So there's really no substitute for the Master Cleanse, which is especially useful for chronic disease sufferers, whether the disease is arthritis or any other autoimmune disorder. If I were ever diagnosed with a chronic disease, the first thing I would do would be a Master Cleanse.

A note of caution: As with the healing process, when you do a cleanse, you may feel worse before you feel better. The early days of the cleanse are usually the hardest; you may not feel good because, as the toxins leave your body, you may experience a series of flu-like symptoms: slight fever, headache (especially if you are used to consuming caffeine), or nausea. You can even develop rashes. These are all just signs of toxins leaving the body and that's exactly what you want. Typically, the more symptoms you experience, the more toxins you have in your body. So if you go through a cleanse and you feel really sick doing it, that just proves that you really needed to do it because there were a lot of toxins built up in your body.

Another great thing about this cleanse is that it is an excellent way to break a bad habit or a bad pattern. If, for instance, you want to break the habit of drinking coffee, there's no better way than to do a cleanse. When you're on the cleanse, obviously, you can't drink any coffee and by doing that you'll see you'll be able to break your addiction to coffee quite easily. Why? Because as you go through the cleanse, you have more energy. You actually have more energy than you would if you drank coffee to begin with. Patients who do the cleanse realize this, and then they just lose their need for coffee. It works for alcohol or any other bad habit. The number-one way to eliminate a bad habit is to stop doing it, and the Master Cleanse provides a framework in which to do that.

My recommendations to arthritic patients who are overweight and have poor diets is to do a seven or ten-day Master Cleanse. It is a lot easier for them to change their diet because they've just gone through a rapid transformation as a result of the fast. They'll be feeling more energetic and they'll be feeling healthier than they have in a long time, if not ever. It's a lot easier to stick to a healthy diet when you're already feeling better and functioning at a much higher level. Actually, as soon as you come off the fast and you start eating again, you'll see how food affects how you feel. As soon as you start eating food again, you lose that euphoric feeling that you had while you were fasting.

Then as time goes on—and this is typical of human nature—you will start to go off course a little bit by returning to some of your old habits. If that happens, all you do is another Master Cleanse. It doesn't have to be a ten-day fast; you could do a three day or a five-day or a seven-day fast, whatever it takes to break those habits again and get you back on track. Overall, the cleanse is a great way to stay on track, stay focused, and keep those habits at bay. As I said earlier, you can think of it as hitting the reset button.

Did I mention it is a great way to lose weight? Obviously, you will lose a significant amount of weight when you are on the cleanse. When I do a 7 to 10-day cleanse, I lose around 10 to 12 pounds. After a few days, I will gain back a couple of pounds, but for the most part, the weight stays off. The benefits you get from the doing the cleanse are magnified when you exercise while on the cleanse, especially if you sweat a lot. The extra calories you burn will enhance your weight loss and the sweating will enhance your detox because sweat is a major way your body releases toxins. Of course, if you go back to eating unhealthy food after the cleanse, the weight will come back. You can keep the weight off by eating healthy food and exercising, but if, after six months or so, you are gaining weight, the fastest way to lose those extra pounds is to do another cleanse. No one said staying healthy would be easy. If it were, 60 percent of the American population wouldn't be overweight.

Warning: When doing the cleanse you cannot take any over the counter or prescription drugs. Doing so could damage your liver because you are not consuming any food. So you must check with your MD to make sure you can stop taking your meds for a limited time.

THE YEAST ISSUE: CANDIDA

Candida albicans is a yeast that can cause a fungus overgrowth in the body. While candida is a common intestinal yeast that everyone has, it becomes a problem when it grows out of control and begins to wreak havoc on the human body. A candida overgrowth has been linked to just about every autoimmune disease, especially diseases with no etiology or no known cause. Many medical doctors are not trained to diagnose a candida problem. They don't know how to test for it, and many times they don't even know to look for it. So typically, patients who have health issues that nobody seems to be able to diagnose usually have, at the very root, a candida problem. The reasons why candida begins to grow out of control are varied, but there are probably three very powerful causes: long-term antibiotic use; steroid use, such as cortisone injections or asthma inhalers; and long-term contraceptive use.

People who have health problems that doctors are unable to help most likely have a candida problem, especially if one of the aforementioned risk factors applies to them. When the candida yeast grows out of control, it starts to manifest itself in different parts of the body. It frequently likes to hang out in joints, such as a knee joint, hip joint, or a shoulder joint. When it does that, it will colonize and start to release toxins called microtoxins that cause a lot of different problems in the body including, but not limited to, the following:

- digestive symptoms such as abdominal pain, acid reflux, belching, bloating, colitis, constipation, Crohn's disease, diarrhea, distended abdomen, food cravings, indigestion, leaky gut syndrome, nausea, heartburn
- anal itching
- thrush
- weight gain
- inability to lose weight
- mental symptoms such as anxiety, ADHD, autism, confusion, depression, dizziness, foggy thinking, hyperactivity, irritability, learning problems, memory loss, migraine/headaches, mood swings, panic, poor concentration, unexplained anger
- other symptoms such as acne, skin irritation, loss of sex drive, fatigue, core throat, joint pain

The symptoms vary from person to person and can fluctuate in severity. There are hundreds of different symptoms ranging from depression to irregular heartbeat. But some of the most common signs or symptoms are abdominal gas, bloating, fatigue, problems with memory, flu-like symptoms, acid reflux, chronic sinus problems, headaches, and even chronic dental problems. In my experience, the most effective way to treat candida is through the Master Cleanse. I'm speaking from experience: I have a candida problem. As a child, I was on long-term antibiotics that destroyed my immune system and I developed candida. As an adult I had to find a cure for it on my own because no doctor could tell me what was happening to me. The reason why the Master Cleanse works is because candida feeds on the foods that we eat, particularly sugar. It loves sugar and a lot of our diets are high in sugar. Even when you eat complex carbohydrates such as rice, cereals, or pastas, the body rapidly converts them to sugar and that's exactly what candida will feed on. When the candida hangs out in the joints, as described above, it will cause inflammation and you begin to experience arthritic-type pain. A lot of times, just by knowing that candida could be a problem and by doing a Master Cleanse and getting the candida under control, you can alleviate a lot of arthritic-type symptoms.

A side note: once you do a cleanse and get the yeast under control, it is possible for the yeast to grow back. Unfortunately, it's going to be a continuing problem because if you go back and start eating the diet you had before you were aware of the candida, the candida can definitely return.

It's an ongoing issue but one that can easily be dealt with by doing a cleanse on a regular basis. As I said, I speak from experience. For me, doing a cleanse twice a year helps keep the candida at bay. For other people once a year may be enough, depending on the severity of symptoms and how strictly they adhere to an anticandida diet. I would rather eat and drink foods I enjoy and do two cleanses a year, but some people who don't want to do a cleanse can often adhere to an anticandida diet and eliminate the candida problem.

Another important point is that candida makes it very difficult to lose weight. Arthritic patients who try to drop weight find it very difficult to do. That's exactly what happened to me. At one time I wanted to lose about 10 pounds, just an inch or two around my waist. I was doing an hour of cardio a day, six days a week, but I wasn't dropping a pound of weight. I was very disappointed and frustrated because I was doing all this aerobic activity and I wasn't dropping any weight. I eventually learned that candida was the issue, and now my weight is stable and my waist size is the same as it was in high school. Once you control the candida, a lot of times the weight you are trying to lose will just drop off. If the candida stays at bay, those pounds will usually stay off. For those of you who want to try to self-diagnose: many times people with candida will develop little red blood blisters over their body. It is estimated that 80 percent of the population has a candida problem and I see many patients who have these little red blood blisters on their body. When I ask patients about them, they always tell me they just showed up out of the blue. People are not born with these blisters. I believe they develop from the microtoxins the colonies of candida release in the body. If you notice red blisters on your body that you where not born with, it means, unfortunately, you have a candida problem, especially if you have some nagging health issues that don't seem to go away. If you have any type of arthritis, a candida problem could be causing some of your symptoms. If you are finding it difficult to lose weight with diet and exercise, candida is likely to blame as well. You cannot expect conventional physicians to find and cure candida because they are not trained to treat this condition. I would not recommend seeing your MD for this type of issue because you will undergo unnecessary testing and you will be misdiagnosed. If you think you may have a candida problem, call my office, and I will be able to help you myself, or I can recommend you to a specialist who can. You can find my contact information in the back of the book. This has been a very brief description of candida, for there are entire books published on this subject, but I wanted to inform readers that candida can contribute to symptoms of arthritis, which may be controlled by addressing the candida problem.

In your Corner: Omega-3 fatty acids (eicosapentaenoic acid and docosahexaenoic acid)—one of the best ways I know for patients to lower inflammation in their bodies is to take high doses of omega-3 fatty acids. A lot of research demonstrates the value of taking high-dose omega-3 fish oil.

Arichidonic acid is an omega-6 fatty acid. Omega-6 and omega-3 fatty acids are supposed to be in balance with each other. Think of omega 6s as the "bad guys" and omega 3s as the "good guys" because an overabundance of omega 6s leads to chronic inflammation and chronic inflammation leads to disease. As a society, this imbalance has been growing in our bodies for decades. At the turn of the last century, in 1900, the ratio was 4:1 omega 6 to omega 3. Currently the ratio is 25:1. This rise in omega imbalance has been attributed to the increase use of vegetable oil consumption from 2 lb. a year in 1909 to 25 lb. a year in 1985! Many of the chronic inflammatory conditions are made worse due to this fatty acid imbalance. And, ironically, going to your medical doctor could make this condition even worse because an MD will give you some type of NSAID for pain instead of addressing the underlying problem: the fatty acid imbalance. A study published in the *Arthritis & Rheumatism* journal in 2002 found that omega-3 fatty acids are anti-inflammatory and they halt or slow the degenerative and inflammatory factors that contribute to osteoarthritis. They were also shown to reduce pain and inflammation in human arthritic conditions.

Another study, a meta-analysis of the analgesic effects of omega-3 fatty acids for anti inflammatory joint pain published in the journal *Pain* in 2007 found supplementation of omega 3s for three to four months reduced patient-reported joint pain, the duration of morning stiffness, the number of painful joints, and NSAID consumption. (It's important to note here that a minimum of three months of supplementation with a dose of 2.7 grams/day of EPA and DHA is required to achieve an anti-inflammatory response.) Consuming omega 3 is just another specific thing patients can do to help alleviate the symptoms of arthritis. Again, with arthritis, we want to control weight and inflammation. The omega-3 fatty acid is a very powerful anti-inflammatory and a great substitute for NSAIDs, which is probably the first line of defense conventional physicians will prescribe for their arthritic patients. NSAIDs—Aleve, ibuprofen, and so on—are anti-inflammatories but with dangerous side effects. Omega 3s are great substitutes because they do the same exact thing but with none of the dangerous side effects. Omega 3 is a fatty acid found in high concentrations in coldwater fish such as mackerel, tuna, and cod. But for these omega-3 fish oils to be effective, they need to be taken in high doses. You can't eat enough mackerel or cod or salmon to get the fatty acids you need for a therapeutic effect. So you've got to supplement your diet with fish oils. When buying a fish oil supplement, you want to be sure the product is free of toxins.

Toxins are taken out of supplements through a process called molecular distillation. A lot of distilled or filtered water is used to get all the mercury and the PCBs out of the fish oil. So you can consume large quantities of fish oils without consuming any of the harmful toxins that may have been in them. When it comes to supplementing with fish oils, you should know that not all supplements are created equal. Some are better than others and a lot of that can be seen in the price. You want to read the label and make sure the oils have been filtered properly. You also want the EPA and the DHA to be in a certain ratio. You want the EPA to be in a 2:1 ratio to the DHA. But that's not as important as making sure that you have pharmaceutical-grade fish oil. That will ensure that all the toxins have been taken out of the fish oil. Studies show that you want to take the fish oil in high doses: from 2000 mg up to 5000 mg depending on the severity of your arthritis. I take 3000 mg a day. I would recommend that you start with 3000 mg of fish oil per day and see how you progress. But it's important to start and maintain those high-dose levels because that's what's been tested and found to be effective.

A BLOOD-THINNING ELEMENT

Omega 3s have been shown to be a powerful anti-inflammatory, but they're also very good at thinning the blood. So anybody who takes an aspirin a day to prevent heart attacks may be able to switch the aspirin for fish oil. The fish oil is just as effective a blood thinner as the aspirin but doesn't have the dangerous side effects that are associated with aspirin. The implications for fish oil are wide ranging: it's been shown to treat and help patients not only with inflammatory conditions such as arthritis but also depression, autism, Alzheimer's, and other cognitive impairments or dysfunction. Fish oils have been shown to be effective because the DHA in them is actually brain food. In fact, most of the brain is made up of the fatty acid DHA (docosahexaenoic acid).

CONTROLLING PAIN WITH OMEGA 3

In April 2006 *Surgical Neurology* reported a study done to see how fish oils acted as an anti-inflammatory compared to NSAID drugs for pain. The study involved 250 patients who suffered from chronic neck or back pain. They had been using daily doses of NSAIDs. They took 1200 mg per day of the omega-3 essential fatty acids. After 75 days of taking high doses of omega 3s, 59 percent of the patients stopped taking the prescription drugs for their pain, and 88 percent said they were pleased enough with the outcome that they plan to continue using the fish oils. No significant adverse effects were reported. Fish oils taken in a high dose have been proven to reduce inflammation, lower your risk for heart disease, reduce pain levels, and help reduce cognitive impairments—all without dangerous side effects—making high-dose fish oil a superior alternative to prescriptions or over-the-counter drugs. If you are going to take pain medications, or NSAID medications for your arthritis, you might as well get the same benefit, without the dangerous side effects associated with NSAIDs, by taking fish oils instead. It makes a lot more sense, but I'm sure the drug companies won't approve.

A WORD ABOUT ARTHRITIS SUPPLEMENTS

There is solid scientific evidence showing that glucosamine and chondroitin sulfate can help improve joint function and reduce pain associated with osteoarthritis.

Glucosamine helps with OA because it has the ability to rebuild damaged cartilage. It stimulates the production of collagen and proteoglycans while at the same time reducing cartilage breakdown. Proteoglycans, collagen, and water are the three building blocks of healthy cartilage. Proteoglycans are essential for cartilage because they attract and hold many times their weight in water. The collagen is what provides the framework for cartilage and holds all the proteoglycans in place.

Chondroitin sulfate is similar to glucosamine sulfate in that they both help build proteoglycans, but chondroitin is unique because it helps attract fluid into the proteoglycan molecules. This is why it is recommended to take both glucosamine and chondroitin together because they work synergistically.

In my experience, these supplements tend to work best in the early stages of arthritis. Their effectiveness seems to diminish with the more advanced cases of OA. If you are reading this and you are 45 or younger, these supplements have a greater chance of helping you. But if you are 65 or older, I would not expect much improvement with these supplements.

If they can help you, I would recommend taking both glucosamine and chondroitin sulfate for 90 days at 1500 mg for glucosamine and 800 mg of chondroitin sulfate daily. If after 90 days you don't realize any improvement, it is safe to say that continued use will not provide any additional benefit and you can discontinue their use.

Due to ample scientific proof of their effectiveness and safety, glucosamine and chondroitin sulfate should be the first line of defense against OA. Why give a toxic and dangerous drug to patients as a first line of defense when these supplements are proven to be safer and more effective, especially as all physicians take an oath to "first do no harm" when they are awarded their license to practice medicine?

When was the last time your doctor recommended you take a supplement? Probably never, right? The question you have to ask yourself is why. If science proves natural supplements are safer and superior to drugs, why are doctors not recommending them? Because drug companies cannot patent a naturally occurring substance. If they can't patent it, they can't corner the market and make a ton of money from the product. Just like anything else in our society, if you want to find the answer to something, just follow the money.

EXERCISE: WHAT'S BEST

When it comes to arthritis and doing home care for arthritis-type pain, exercise is a very beneficial. Exercise has been proven by many scientific studies to be very good for the body in general but especially for osteoarthritis. The body likes motion and it heals with motion, so anyone with arthritis, or anyone who wants to prevent OA, should incorporate some type of physical exercise into his or her regimen. Patients can use exercise to increase the success of laser therapy, improve their arthritis symptoms overall, and also prevent arthritis from occurring in the first place. One of the reasons why exercise is necessary for arthritis is the fact that cartilage is avascular (no blood supply). Without blood supply, cartilage must get its nourishment from synovial fluid through a process called imbibition. For the cartilage to imbibe synovial fluid, the joints must move. Take the knee joint, for example. When you walk, the cartilage will work much like a sponge. With every step you take, the fluid will be pressed in and out of the cartilage. This movement of the synovial fluid is how the cartilage stays nourished and healthy. Any prolonged inactivity will cause the cartilage to further weaken and break down due to the lack of proper nourishment. This is the reason why exercise is important for people before and after they develop any type of arthritic symptom. The problem is arthritis symptoms usually take years to develop, So some patients won't realize they have arthritis until the symptoms develop, but once they do, it may be painful to exercise. In other words, some patients don't get a warning sign they have arthritis to motivate them to exercise. Others, however, may get an early warning sign, usually in the form of joint stiffness. Those patients who develop stiffness first, without joint pain, should take that as a warning sign and start an exercise program, because if they wait, it is just a matter of time until painful symptoms develop, making exercise intolerable. The first step in starting an exercise program is to undergo a physical exam, especially if you are a male over forty years old or a female over fifty years old, and anyone of any age who is considered high risk should undergo a medical exam to make sure exercise will be safe. I know the vast majority of people will not take the time or expense to get medical clearance to start an exercise program, but it is important not just for the medical clearance; it is a great way to obtain baseline measurements of blood pressure, body fat, and blood lipids that can quantify patients' progress—other than monitoring pain levels—during their exercise program. Some people find it difficult to stick with an exercise program. So I would recommend starting with a simple walking program, which will allow you to avoid the costs of buying equipment or joining a gym before you are confident you will enjoy exercise and will want to continue. Walking is a good way to start because you can do it outside or inside and you probably won't need any guidance on how to walk properly. Everyone knows how to walk, but many people don't know how to exercise properly. So they will have to rely on a health professional to show them what to do and how to do it properly. You can spend money on a more advanced exercise program after you start walking and are so encouraged by the benefits that you will want to stick with the exercise program. Another reason walking is good for OA is that it offers low impact activity, aids weight loss, and provides nourishment for weight-bearing articular cartilage. Walking is safe for just about everybody. The only precaution I have is to not walk through pain. If it hurts to walk, that is a sign to stop; continuing to walk through pain may cause more damage to your joints. If you are in pain when you walk, try riding a stationary bike. The other precaution to take is to walk on a smooth, even surface, such as a sidewalk or track. Walking on rough surfaces creates uneven stress on the cartilage of weight-bearing joints, which can cause further damage to the cartilage. As long as you don't walk through pain and walk on a smooth, flat surface, you will find walking to be an enjoyable and worthwhile activity. Walking is a low-intensity exercise. Therefore it can be done on a daily basis and that is what I would recommend, but I would walk every other day to start and increase it to every day as you get in better shape. For most people the goal would be to walk for an hour a day on a daily basis at a brisk pace. Once you are comfortable walking and want to increase your exercise program, you can begin to incorporate weight lifting into your routine. Weight training will allow you to increase muscle mass, bone density, and weight loss. Weight training isn't just for young people. Weight training has been shown to increase muscle mass and strength for the elderly. People well into their eighties can improve their muscle mass and bone density with weight training. I know this firsthand because I did an internship at Tufts University Research Center on Aging in Boston, Massachusetts, during my senior year at the University of Massachusetts. During my internship I was involved in a number of different studies and all of them involved strength training and the elderly. I learned many different things, but the one lasting impression I took from that internship is watching patients in their eighties working out with weights. It was great to see them lifting weights, but what was more impressive was seeing their before and after muscle biopsies. All the patients' biopsies I looked at showed an increase in muscle mass! That internship and the research they were doing there at Tufts University proved that anyone can increase his or her muscle mass and bone density no matter what age he or she is. For anyone reading this in advanced age: do not think you are too old to exercise because science says you are never too old to experience all the benefits weight training offers. What is important to note about the benefits of weight training is that it is not just about getting stronger; it is about the increased functional capacity an elderly person can develop. The major reason most elderly people move into retirement homes is because they can no longer care for themselves at home. They may not be able to climb stairs, lift a laundry basket, or climb in and out of the shower. All these things can be improved with strength training. What I want people reading this to understand is that they are never too old to get stronger, and by getting stronger, many people may be able to not only reduce their arthritis symptoms but also remain independent and keep living in their own home. I have listed the benefits of exercise specifically for OA, but exercise does so many good things to the body, I would be doing the reader an injustice by not listing all of the health benefits.

Exercise does the following:

- Increases muscle mass: The more muscle you have the greater amount of calories you burn at rest. The calories you burn at rest come from fat, so you will burn more fat while you sleep. This relates to better body composition, more lean muscle, and less fat;
- Increases bone density: denser bone is stronger bone and stronger bones help prevent bone fractures;
- Increases immune function: better immune function equals better protection from sickness and disease;
- Improves sleep and relaxation: during sleep your body repairs and regenerates;
- Reduces stress: stress is a major contributor to chronic disease;
- Improves self-image: Losing weight and inches help people feel better about themselves. According to Dr. Maxwell Maltz and his best-selling book *Psycho-Cybernetics*, people's success is determined by their self-image. If you can change your self-image, you can change your life;

- Improves intestinal peristalsis: Peristalsis is the movement of food through the digestive tract. This allows better digestion and regularity;
- Improves blood lipids: exercise lowers bad (LDL) cholesterol and raises good (HDL) cholesterol;
- Increases stroke volume: Stroke volume is the amount of blood you heart sends out per beat. Increasing the amount of blood per beat increases the efficiency of your heart because your heart will be able to get the required amount of blood to the body in less beats;
- Prevents diabetes: increased insulin sensitivity is why you can just about guarantee you will not develop diabetes if you exercise on a regular basis;
- Fights depression: Beta-endorphins are the feel-good hormones your body releases during exercise. These hormones are more powerful than morphine and are powerful against depression. It is almost impossible not to feel good after exercise;
- Prevents cardiovascular disease: heart attacks and stroke rates are reduced with exercise;
- Increases libido (increased sex drive);
- Improves blood pressure;
- Improves balance (through improved proprioception and muscle coordination).

There are many different exercise types and routines you can do today. You can work out at home, join a gym, do Pilates, yoga, Tai Chi, swimming, biking, or walking, to name a few. There are all kinds of different things you do to reduce or even prevent OA. There is not one routine that works best for everybody because people have different likes and dislikes. For example, some people enjoy working

out at home for the convenience, while others may enjoy the cama-
raderie of working out in a gym. What it comes down to is finding
what you enjoy doing and building an exercise routine around that.
I think it is obvious that the more you enjoy doing something the
greater chance you have of being consistent and successful in your
exercise routine. My goal in writing this chapter is not to show you
how to exercise or stretch; that is for another book entirely. My goal
is to tell you what science says is the best form of exercise and then
you can take that information and have a health professional design
a program for you or you can do it on your own. Those of you who
are educated in designing exercise programs can use this information and design your own program. But for those of you without
any experience in designing exercise programs, I would advise getting
professional help from a exercise physiologist, chiropractor, physical
therapist, or personal trainer.

In my experience medical doctors are not trained in exercise and
therefore should not be counted on to prescribe exercise routines.
Again, their focus has always been on prescribing drugs for every
ailment they see in their practice and because of that, they are very
limited in other areas of treatment.

All exercise can be divided in two groups: aerobic and anaerobic.
The only difference between the two is oxygen. Aerobic exercise uses
oxygen and anaerobic does not. The ability to use oxygen during
exercise is directly related to the intensity of the workout. With a
low-intensity exercise such as walking our body is using predominately fat as energy because there are many fat reserves in the body,
and fat is not as efficient a fuel for energy as carbohydrates. So when
the body is engaged in low-intensity activity, the rate at which the
body needs to generate energy is slow, which allows sufficient time
for the body to convert fat to energy. On the other hand, with a

high-intensity exercise such as sprinting, energy is needed at a much faster rate, so carbohydrates must be the energy source because they convert quickly to energy. In other words, your body has two main fuels to make energy. One is carbohydrates (or sugar) and the other is fat. Those two substances provide the energy to move or work out. You can look at sugar as the high-octane gas that you use to fill your car, and fat can be compared to diesel fuel. You'll get more mileage out of the diesel, but its efficiency is not very good relative to sugar. Sugar is very fast acting and better for high-intensity activity, but you can't use it for very long, usually only for seconds. You can get a lot more out of burning fat, as far as calories go, than you can out of sugar. The disparity between fat and carbohydrates is that you only get four calories of energy out of one gram of carbohydrates, but you can get nine calories of energy out of one gram of fat. Because the human body has an abundance of stored fat and a very limited amount of stored carbohydrates, the body uses fat predominately for energy and only uses carbohydrates for high-intensity exercise. I think there is a lot of confusion about what type of exercise is best: aerobic or anaerobic. The confusion isn't just among the general public; I think most health professionals are confused as well. When I say "best," I mean which type of exercise provides the most benefit in the most efficient way. Science says anaerobic exercise burns more calories overall and also more fat compared to aerobic activity. The most appealing part of this type of exercise is that you burn more calories and more fat IN LESS TIME! In today's fast-paced world, where the most common excuse for not exercising is not having enough time, anaerobic exercise solves the time problem because it can be done in a fraction of the time that aerobic exercise takes.

Let me give you an example. Say, for instance, we have two people exercising for 30 minutes. Person A does aerobic exercise at an intensity of 60 percent of the maximum heart rate while person B does interval training or sprint training at an intensity of 60 percent maximum heart rate. But then, every few minutes, person B will increase that to about 85 percent for a very short period and then return to the lower intensity. So person A would just do a very steady state, probably like a very slow jog, for the full 30 minutes. Person B would do that slow jog but then change to a really rapid sprint for a short interval before going back down to a slow jog, followed by another really fast sprint before returning, again, to that slow jog.

What studies have found is that after 30 minutes, person A burned 200 calories total, 60 percent of which was from fat and 40 percent was from sugar. Therefore person A burned 120 total units of fat and 80 units of sugar. Person B, who exercised at the higher intensity, burned 50 percent from fat and 50 percent from sugar. So the percentage was about equal as far as fats compared to sugar, but person B burned 300 calories total. So person B burned 150 units of fat and 150 units of sugar. You can see that person B burned more energy and also more fat compared to person A, even though a lower percentage of the total energy was coming from fat. This is a very common misconception: people believe that if you do a low-intensity exercise, such as a very slow jog or even a fast walk, you're going to burn more fat than if you do a sprint.

That's not true because the slow group will burn a higher percentage of their calories from fat when they're at a slow pace. But when you're sprinting, you're burning so much more energy that the total amount of fat you burn will be greater than the slower group, even though the percentage of fat you're burning during that sprint is less, percentage-wise, than that of the aerobic group. So relatively speaking it's true, but it's absolutely false, and all you care about are the absolute results. You want to burn more fat. You don't care what percentage of your energy is coming from fat at the time. When you're done, you want to be burning more fat than less fat. That's what you get with the anaerobic exercise; you actually burn more fat than you do with aerobic exercise. So it's actually better for patients to do short duration burst training or interval training than it is to just go at a slow steady rate on, say, a treadmill or a stationary bike.

A cautionary note: while technically speaking sprinting is the best form of exercise to burn calories and fat, it may not be suited for all fitness types. I wanted to share this information with you so you would know that for those who have the ability to sprint, sprinting is the best form of exercise. However, for those who do not have the ability to sprint, regular aerobic activity will suffice.

AN EASIER WAY: THE X-ISER®

Now that you know how important it is to do interval training, the question is where do you do it? To sprint safely, most people have to go to the track or find stadium steps to run up and down. However, there is now a product on the market that can help you got that level of intensity safely at home. It's called the X-iser. It is a small portable device that looks like a stepper machine. It only weighs 14 pounds and it's designed to allow you to get an anaerobic workout using the sprinter. You can have it in your office or you can have it in your house. It doesn't take up much space and it's so light and small you can take it anywhere. The beauty of this thing is you can use it in about 120th of the time you would spend doing an aerobic exercise such as jogging or walking, and you'll burn more calories and more fat, and you'll also build more muscle mass.

You can buy the machine online. The X-iser is a particularly great product for patients with painful knees, hips, or back. It's usually tough for them to do jogging or running, but this machine has no impact. It doesn't hurt the joints, so it's safe for patients with arthritis. And it's going to increase not only the fat loss but muscle mass and also bone mass at the same time. It's good too for the elderly population because it helps them improve their balance and their coordination.

Here's another study to consider. It was done in 1994 and reported in the *Journal of Metabolism*. The study tracked two groups of people who were undergoing different modes of exercise. Group 1 did all aerobic training for a period of 20 weeks while group 2 did 15 weeks of high-intensity interval training. So group 2 had five less weeks of training than group 1.

The researchers wanted to see how each program would affect body fat and metabolism. The results showed that the aerobic group burned 48 percent more calories than the interval group over the course of the study. However, despite the big caloric disadvantage, the interval group enjoyed nine times the loss of subcutaneous fat. Remarkably, the resting levels of 3-hydroxyacyl-coenzyme A, an enzyme marker of fat burning, were significantly elevated in the interval group, which they didn't experience in the aerobic group. The interval group trained for five less weeks than the aerobic group; they had shorter workouts and yet they far exceeded the aerobic group in fat burning at rest and during exercise. That study just proves the effectiveness that anaerobic exercise has over aerobic exercise when it comes to fat burning. That's one of the main things you want to accomplish with an exercise program, especially as it pertains to controlling arthritis and your weight. There's no better way to do that than to burn more fat. So burn as much fat as you can in the shortest amount of time; that's what the anaerobic X-iser does for patients.

Who wouldn't want to exercise in half the time and burn more fat? I'd rather spend 15 minutes sprinting than 30 minutes or 45 minutes on the treadmill. It's just the best of both worlds and solves the most common excuse for not exercising: not having enough time.

STRETCHING

Stretching is probably the most neglected aspect of an exercise routine, but that in no way reflects the importance of stretching in keeping joints healthy. As I mentioned earlier, the cartilage in your joints is avascular, so the cartilage must get nourishment through movement or inbibition. In a normal healthy joint, getting proper nutrition is easy, but if the cartilage begins to break down or there is a muscle imbalance, that process of imbibition is inhibited, leaving your joints malnourished. This is why stretching is important to any exercise program but especially for arthritis. If joint stiffness develops, that joint loses its full range of motion. The cartilage in the area where the joint can no longer move will become malnourished and will cause further decay and damage to the cartilage, making symptoms worse

Stretching can help restore the normal range of motion in a joint. The joints in our bodies are surrounded by muscles and these muscles are there to move the joint. Normally, the muscles oppose each other and work synergistically together, in balance, but frequently, a muscle imbalance develops. Take the elbow joint, for instance. The biceps muscle flexes the arm while the triceps muscle opposes the biceps and extends the arm. Ideally, these two muscles oppose each other equally, leaving a joint with a full range of motion. Once a muscle imbalance develops, the joint no longer has its full range of motion. If the triceps becomes weak compared to the biceps, the arm will no longer fully extend because the biceps is overpowering the triceps, pulling the arm in flexion. A very common joint to develop an imbalance is the hip joint. The muscles in the back of the thigh (hamstrings) are made of three separate muscles: the semitendinosus, semimembranosus, and the biceps femoris. The hamstrings are prone to becoming tight while the muscles on the front of the thigh, the quadriceps (rectus femoris, vastus lateralis, vastus intermedius, and vastus medialis) usually become weak. When this occurs, the weak muscles (quadriceps) must be strengthened and the strong or tight muscles (hamstrings) must be stretched to correct the imbalance. If this muscle imbalance continues, the hip joint will lose its full range of motion, leaving the cartilage damaged, due to the lack of nourishment. I hope that makes sense and you can understand how important stretching is for healthy joints. Ideally, stretching should be done before and after exercise. For best results stretching should be done when the muscles are warm and full of blood. It is best to do some light activity before the stretch. If you are going to stretch the legs, it is best to walk or ride a stationary bike for 5–10 minutes, or if you are going to stretch the shoulder, you could do one set of shoulder presses with a light weight before you stretch the shoulder. A muscle that is warm is more pliable and will be able to stretch better than a muscle that is cold. Once the muscles are warmed up and it's time to stretch, it is most important to stretch slowly in a controlled manner, with no bouncy or jerky movements. I would recommend doing a stretch three times and holding each stretch for 10–20 seconds before and after each workout.

Chapter 6

PAYING FOR YOUR TREATMENT

HOW TO AFFORD THE BEST CARE

Not too long ago, I had a conversation with a patient who was spending money out of pocket to pay for his laser treatments. He told me that he wanted to use his insurance to pay for his knee replacement surgery, which would be free to him. I asked him how much he was paying every month in insurance premiums, and he said that he and his wife pay a total of $800 a month. Obviously that surgery isn't free. That comes to $9600 a year they're paying in insurance premiums, and his premiums may even go up after he has that expensive knee-replacement surgery. Moreover, in addition to the insurance premium and depending on which state patients live in and which type of insurance coverage they have, there will be hidden costs such as co-pays and deductibles. For instance, Medicare patients living in New Hampshire would pay $4250 out of pocket for a knee replacement. My laser treatments don't even cost what someone would pay in New Hampshire for a knee replacement even with Medicare!

The other issue with joint replacements is that all artificial joints need to be replaced at some point because they wear out over time, so you can't call them a cure for arthritis. Maybe they offer a longer-term solution, but they are not a cure.

So my point is that even though insurance may cover much of the cost of a surgery, most patients will still have out-of-pocket expenses.

Plus, you have all the obvious risks of surgery, and a long rehabilitation with a hip or knee replacement. You go through all that and ten years down the road, they tell you, "Yeah, your replacement is wearing out; you're going to have to have that replaced," and then you have out-of-pocket expenses again.

I just wanted to put that out there so a patient reading this book can understand that even with insurance, medical treatment isn't free. However, there are options when it comes to paying for care and being able to afford the best treatment possible.

HEALTH SAVINGS ACCOUNTS

Just as they don't know about laser therapy for arthritis, a lot of people don't know that health savings accounts exist. Health savings accounts and high-deductible insurance plans became available in 2002, right around when Congress changed the laws to allow them. Typically, insurance covers sickness care. If you get sick, you go to the doctor who will give you drugs or some other form of treatment, and insurance will cover that visit.

But insurance coverage for alternative care treatments such as chiropractic is very limited. Now, that has changed. Now with these health savings accounts, people can pay for all different types of wellness care such as chiropractic, laser therapy, acupuncture or massage and get the same tax benefits as they would for conventional health care.

It's a much better deal for patients and even employers. In 1980, 80 percent of employers covered their employees' health care. Today, that number is dwindling. Less than 60 percent of jobs now offer health-care benefits. And, as is typical with job-related health insurance, if you lose your job, you lose your insurance.

Because of that, over two million people in the United States have filed for bankruptcy because of medical bills. Most of these families had traditional health insurance when they became ill, but when they couldn't work, they lost their job and their health insurance. Then they were stuck with these huge medical bills. Without any income, they went into bankruptcy. One of the main benefits of opting out of employer-sponsored group-health-insurance plans and buying individualized health insurance is that you wont lose your insurance if you get sick and lose your job plus it qualifies you to open a health savings account.

HEALTH SAVINGS VS. FLEXIBLE SPENDING ACCOUNTS

I mentioned a health savings account, but other similar plans may be more familiar, such as flexible spending accounts. FSAs were around before health savings accounts and they're similar, but the advantage with the health savings account is that you don't lose the benefits at the year's end. With the flexible spending account, you can use the money for health-related expenses tax free, but you lose the money you don't use by the end of the year. That is a big, big problem with that type of plan, but now, with health savings accounts, whatever you don't use at the end of the year is carried over to the following year. The beauty of HSAs is that they're triple tax advantaged. You don't pay any tax when you put money in; you don't pay any tax when you take money out to pay for a health-related expense, and you don't pay any tax on the money that accumulates while it's in the health savings account. Even when you reach the age of 65 and retire, you can pull all the money out. You don't have to use it for a medical expense and you don't pay any tax at that point, which is a big advantage. Even with 401k plans, when you hit retirement age and you pull money out, you have to pay income taxes on that money. But with the health savings account, you don't pay any income tax once you reach the retirement age and pull money out. Before retirement age, you don't pay any taxes as long as you're taking the money out for a covered health-care expense.

Because of this clear benefit, health savings accounts probably represent the biggest change in health care and even retirement care since Social Security and Medicare. When HSAs first became available, more than two million Americans opened up accounts. Let's say a typical single male who has employer-sponsored health insurance with a high premium and low deductible switches to a high-deductible insurance plan. He's going to save probably 40 percent in premium payments because of the higher deductible. The money he saves can then be put into a health savings account, which will cover the deductible if he becomes sick and he needs to use the insurance.

THE NUMBERS IN YOUR FAVOR

Let's say a patient spends $5000 a year for traditional, low-deductible health insurance. If that patient raised the annual deductible by $2000, he or she could reduce the annual premium payments by $2000 or more, which could be placed in the health savings account as an investment in that patient's wellness care. This gives the patient more control over how his or her money is spent. People need to be more proactive about their health care. Typical traditional insurance only pays for drugs, surgery, or physical therapy. With the health savings account, patients can now spend their tax-free dollars on wellness expenses such as chiropractic care, acupuncture, laser therapy, dental work, and even cancer screenings, this is just a partial list there is a long list of qualified medical expenses on the IRS website

ANOTHER OPTION: FINANCING YOUR LASER THERAPY

In my office we also offer patients the option to finance their care. This is best for patients who don't have credit cards and/or can't afford to pay for their care up front. We use an outside finance company called Care Credit. You will find many dentists, chiropractors, and even plastic surgeons offering financing through Care Credit, which is a subsidiary of General Electric (GE). The greatest benefit to the patient besides being able to stretch the payments out is the fact that Care Credit charges no interest as long as the patient doesn't make a late payment and the balance is paid off in 12 months. I pay for the service; that's why Care Credit can afford to offer no-interest payment plans. Just a word of caution: if you make one late payment or fail to pay off the balance in 12 months, Care Credit will charge you interest at a rate of around 24 percent. This is a good program, but you need to make sure you pay the balance off within 12 months and never make a late payment. For patients who can't afford to pay off their care in 12 months, Care Credit also has interest-bearing payment plans with durations of 24 and 60 months; the interest rate at the time of this writing is 14.9 percent.

However you decide to handle your care, remember that even when you use your health insurance for medical treatment, there will be an out-of-pocket cost in premiums, co-pays, and deductibles. But you can actually save money in the long run by having laser therapy. It's not just about saving money, though; it's about enjoying higher quality of life. Money becomes irrelevant when laser therapy is able to give patients their life back. I'm sure all those who have ever had to give up something they love because of pain would pay just about any amount of money to be able to enjoy that activity again. I have had so many patients—too many to list here—who were able to get back to doing things they enjoy because they underwent my laser therapy program. Anyone reading this who is in pain, please take the time to read all of the testimonials provided in this book. You will be inspired by all of the different things patients were able to get back to doing because of my laser therapy program. I remember a particular patient telling me she was contemplating suicide due to the chronic pain she had been suffering for more than twenty years. Luckily, she didn't go to such an extreme because now that she has finished her laser treatment, she is almost 100 percent pain-free. That is the power of my laser therapy; it offers you the best chance to become free of chronic pain and get your life back because no one should suffer in pain when my laser program has made so many patients better.

Conclusion

Arthritis is the leading cause of chronic pain and disability in the United States, accounting for 17 percent of all disability nationwide. Not only does arthritis cause pain and disability in large numbers of people, the costs associated with treating it, about $15 billion in direct medical costs, are staggering. If you include lost work productivity, the costs climb to $83 billion every single year. The primary reason arthritis causes so much pain and disability and costs so much is due to the very limited and ineffective treatment options conventional physicians offer. Not only are their treatments ineffective, but they often result in dangerous side effects that cause more pain and disability and lead to more costs. The side effects might be worth the risk if the drugs provided long-term pain relief, but they do not. All of the available conventional medical treatments for osteoarthritis are palliative, meaning they are only meant to help relieve the symptoms temporarily.

Let me go over these conventional medical treatments for arthritis again because I think it is important for you to understand that no matter how many different conventional doctors you consult, or how many times you go back to them, you are only going to be offered one of four treatment options: drugs, corticosteroid injections, surgery, or physical therapy. Even if you have hip or knee replacement surgery, it is not considered a cure because these artificial joints have to be replaced in 10–15 years. Medical treatments for arthritis not only don't fix the problem, they actually make it worse. Consider, for example, a patient who is taking an NSAID drug daily to deal with arthritis pain and the NSAID causes a bleeding ulcer. Now that patient has another medical condition requiring more treatments and additional costs. In fact, up to 30 percent of patients taking NSAIDs develop gastrointestinal symptoms, resulting in 103,000 hospitalizations a year.

Problems from spinal surgery occur so often they actually had to give the condition a name. Doctors coined the term failed back surgery syndrome, which refers to patients who had spinal surgery but still have chronic back or neck pain. I would guess that would be a red flag if a certain procedure fails so often they have to give it a name. Come to think of it, there is a name for all of the different side effects that conventional medical treatments cause. When a doctor gives a prescription drug or performs a procedure that causes undesired side effects, the term for such problems is *iatrogenic* (pronounced i-*at*-tro-*genic*), meaning "doctor caused."

According to a landmark study in *The Journal of the American Medical Association, iatrogenic* problems are the third leading cause of death in the United States! I guess that would be another red flag to be aware of when you go to the hospital or your local conventional doctor. I want to be very clear: conventional doctors are not intentionally harming patients. This is not a personal attack on conventional medicine. I am just stating the facts and the facts show that conventional doctors' currently available treatment options for arthritis of any type don't provide any cure and many times make matters worse due to the risk of dangerous side effects. I want to be clear on this issue: conventional medicine is not the place to go if you have arthritis pain or numbness. If you are in a car accident or any other severe trauma and need to be put back together, then U.S. conventional medicine is the best. But for the treatment of arthritis it is inadequate at best and I think most conventional doctors realize that. That's why many of them tell their patients they will just have to live with their arthritis pain.

That was acceptable advice prior to 2003. Today, with the availability of the incredible power of the 15 watt class-4 laser, it is terrible advice. Unfortunately, you should not expect your medical doctor to refer you to a doctor like me (e.g., a chiropractor) to get laser therapy. In a perfect health-care system they would, but in our broken, conventional system, chiropractors, or any alternative-care doctors, are seen as competition. That's obviously a shame because it only hurts the patients. A great way to distinguish a good doctor from a bad one is to gauge a conventional doctor's response when you ask him or her about seeking alternative care for the treatment of arthritis. If he or she discourages you from doing so, I would find a new doctor because that is an obvious sign that your doctor is putting his or her interests ahead of yours. I would find a doctor who is happy to send you elsewhere for treatment because that is a sign that your doctor has your best interests in mind. For all the millions of people suffering from arthritis pain, your best treatment option by far is the class-4 15-watt infrared laser.

Osteoarthritis is a disease of the cartilage in your joints. When your cartilage begins to break down or crack, the degenerative process begins, and you will begin to experience joint stiffness, pain, and inflammation. When the cartilage is healthy, the bones in the joint move smoothly with no friction, but when it cracks, the smooth surface becomes rough, thus creating pain and inflammation. My class-4 laser works so well on arthritis pain because the chondrocytes (which are the cartilage cells) are stimulated by the laser to repair themselves and regenerate. In essence, the damaged chondrocytes absorb the most light from the laser and it is this process that allows the damaged cartilage to repair itself and/or rebuild itself into healthy cartilage. I should say that it is *hypothesized* that class-4 laser therapy can repair the damaged cartilage because it has not been proven scientifically. Science has proved that chondrocytes are stimulated by laser therapy and that the stimulation leads to cellular repair and regeneration in a test tube, but no studies have yet been carried out that have specifically tested whether human cartilage is increased after laser therapy treatment. The only way to do that would be to test a group of patients by means of an MRI examination of their cartilage before and after laser treatment.

I don't need to see any study proving the efficacy of laser therapy because I see laser therapy changing people's lives every day. I have had hundreds of patients who have had such bad arthritis in their knees that knee replacement surgery was recommended. These patients had virtually no cartilage. X-rays revealed "bone on bone." Many times these same patients get significant pain relief from my laser therapy and because the pain relief has the potential to last for years, the cartilage must have been affected, otherwise the pain would return soon after treatment had been completed. Conventional doctors for years have criticized nonmedical treatments because there are often no scientific studies to prove their effectiveness. But in no way does that lack of scientific proof mean alternative treatments are fraudulent or ineffective. Chiropractic is the largest alternative medicine specialty and has been in existence over 100 years. Regardless of how much scientific proof there is behind chiropractic, the profession would not have survived this long if it did not help patients—period! The irony of the conventional medicine community calling alternative health-care practitioners unscientific is that only 15 percent of medical procedures are scientifically proved to help patients. That's not a typo: only 15 percent of medical treatments are backed up by science! Does the fact that only 15 percent of medical procedures are backed up by science make conventional medicine scientific? I sure don't think so, especially when I can give you examples of some of the most common surgical procedures done in this country that have been scientifically proved not to work. I'm sure everyone reading this has heard of someone who has had coronary artery bypass surgery (CABG). During this surgery a vein is usually taken from a patient's leg and connected to a clogged coronary artery, bypassing the blockage. Every year, 515,000 of these procedures are performed costing $34 billion. It is one of the most commonly performed surgeries in the country. Unfortunately, there were two large, very well done studies done more than two decades ago that prove coronary bypass surgery does not help patients increase their life span or quality of life: the Veterans Study of 686 patients, published in the *New England Journal of Medicine*; and the Coronary Artery Surgery Study, or CASS study. I can go on and on with a list of examples proving this troubling trend.

In fact, the entire discipline of psychiatry is built upon the lie that depression is caused by a chemical imbalance of serotonin in the brain. It is a lie because it is impossible to measure the levels of serotonin in the human brain. These chemicals are too small to be able to measure, thus making it impossible to determine if there is an imbalance. When you consider the only form of treatment psychiatrists offer to depressed patients is the class of antidepressant drugs called SSRI (selective serotonin reuptake inhibitors), you can see why drug companies and psychiatrists continue to promote these drugs for depression, claiming that depression is caused by this serotonin imbalance. So the drug manufacturers fabricate scientific studies to "prove" depression is caused by a serotonin chemical imbalance in the brain.

Getting back to arthritis treatments, during the 1990s, the commonest surgical procedure done in the United States was arthroscopic knee surgery. Some 650,000 of these procedures were done on a yearly basis with a cost of $5,000 each. If you do the math it comes out to over $3 billion in costs each year. I'm sure those were the good old days for orthopedic surgeons because in 2002 it all came crashing down. On July 11, 2002, a study published in the *New England Journal of Medicine* (NEJM) titled, "A Controlled Trial of Arthroscopic Surgery for Osteoarthritis in the Knee," found that this surgery provided no benefit to patients.

The study was done on 180 patients with arthritis of the knee. The surgery group received standard arthroscopic treatment and the placebo group was subjected to a skin incision without actually having arthroscopic treatment. None of the 180 patients knew which group they were in and the doctors assessing their outcomes were also unaware of which form of treatment the patients had received. The golden standard for scientific studies is a double-blinded placebo controlled study with a large group of patients. This study satisfied all three, making it a very well done scientific study. The patients were studied over a 24-month follow-up period and the patients who received the sham procedure experienced the same results as the patients who had the real procedure done!

During standard arthroscopic surgery, the surgeon will often remove a damaged meniscus and scrape and or file the existing cartilage in an attempt to smooth the damaged cartilage. This scraping and filing is just as much of a trauma to the patient as a fractured leg would be. So, not only does arthroscopic surgery provide no benefit to patients, it actually causes further damage to the cartilage. I bet if you followed the same patients in the study, 5 to 10 years later, you would find their osteoarthritis was worse than the patients who had had the sham procedure.

Earlier in the book I listed trauma to a joint, such as a fracture from a car accident, as a major cause of osteoarthritis. Now you can add arthroscopic surgery to the list of causes. To this day arthroscopic surgery is still being done, though not at the same rate as before. But this still serves as another example of conventional medicine lacking scientific proof for some of the most commonly performed surgical procedures. How the medical community can justify doing these surgeries on patients when they have been scientifically proven not to work is beyond comprehension, especially when you consider coronary bypass surgery has a 3–5 percent mortality rate, meaning thousands of people die every year from the operation. But that is a story for another book. Those who want to learn more can read *Heart Frauds: Uncovering the Biggest Health Scam in History* by Charles McGee, or *The Great American Heart Hoax* by Dr. Michael Ozner, MD.

I hope I have given enough examples proving conventional medicine is far from evidence based, and any attempt by the conventional medicine community to claim laser treatment, or any alternative medicine, is inferior to conventional medicine because it lacks scientific proof is the pot calling the kettle black.

It is quite unfortunate for arthritic patients that conventional doctors do not refer them to alternative treatments, especially since just about all patients seek care from their conventional doctor first, before trying any other type of treatment. Most patients have a blind faith in their conventional medicine practitioner, which, together with the insistence of conventional doctors on keeping patients in their medical system, often leads a patient to surgery before trying safer, more effective treatments first.

One of my goals in writing this book is to change that process, but I can't do it on my own. I need your help. I encourage you to tell as many people as possible about this book and about laser therapy because the more people understand the benefits of laser therapy, the greater chance we have of helping patients get long-lasting relief from arthritis pain and numbness. The reform of health care and reduction of health-care costs can only happen through the efforts of the general public. We can't count on the medical profession to change the way they do business because they would be taking money out of their own pockets. We can't expect the people who make the rules and enact the laws of the current health-care system to change their ways because they are the same people who profit from that system. It is up to us public consumers to become informed patients.

I hope it is apparent by now that the best available treatment for arthritis pain and numbness is the class-4, 15-watt, deep-tissue laser. This laser is not just the best available treatment; it is in a class all by itself. The class-4 laser cannot be compared to any other arthritis treatment because it is the only modality that produces long-term pain relief with zero side effects. I want to drive this point home because many of my patients come to me after trying every imaginable treatment available and they have been told by all these different doctors or therapists that their treatment would be able to get them better. So, naturally, when I tell them that my treatment gives them the best chance to get better, they are skeptical because they have heard it all before and are still in pain. My response to these patients is that you cannot compare class-4 laser therapy to any other treatment because there is no other treatment that stimulates cellular repair and regeneration while simultaneously reducing inflammation, decreasing pain eight different ways, increasing blood flow, and creating new blood vessels (angiogenesis). On top of all those benefits you will be relieved to know that you get all that upside with no downside, as in side effects. I know it sounds too good to be true. If this were a financial investment, my advice would be to stay away from it because in the financial world, investments that sound too good to be true often are. In this case, it sounds too good to be true but it is true. That's the reason 15 watt class-4 laser therapy is revolutionizing the treatment of arthritis pain.

Patient Testimonials

I'm much more mobile than prior to treatment. I'm playing better tennis and some agility has returned. I have little or no pain in the back lower left pelvic area. My left leg is more mobile in its ability to turn left and right. The leg is still slow in walking, but it's better than before the treatment.
—Alma Cirino, age 81

The laser treatments reduced the pain in my very sore left hip. The laser heat seemed to stimulate healing or lower inflammation in my torn hip labrum.
—Andre Wooten, age 63

I can go days without pain, can walk without use of a cane. The greatest improvement is that I have little or no pain, can do most of the things like cooking, cleaning, sewing, and so forth, on a daily basis.
—Betty Y. A., age 83

This treatment has improved my life immensely. My lower back pain that I used to feel daily has gone away completely. My back has a wider range of flexibility and increased muscle strength. I have returned to exercising and feel healthier and happier. I used to have lower back pain while driving so much I disliked driving. I would toss and turn in my sleep because of the discomfort; now I sleep peacefully. At work I can run the register for four hours without the discomfort.
—Caitlin Spidle, age 27

After my first treatment the swelling in my right knee settled to a point where I could kneel down and work again. I can now squat all the way down and work with no pain. I can also work resting on my knees.
—Carl Nagatoshi, age 48

My palm and the first three fingers were numb. The LiteCure laser has helped my nerve that controls the palm and first three fingers. Now I can feel things and do my work around the house and write better. I am very happy there is LiteCure laser in Hawaii.
—**Christina Goya, age 90**

My pain has decreased about 90 percent so far. I am very pleased with the results! Now I am able to sleep through the night without getting up at about three or four in the morning. I am much happier and well rested.
—**Cindy Higa-Dunn, age 47**

My pain in my left leg, tingling—with this treatment I feel so much better. I walk and sleep much more peacefully.
—**Cynthia Kaleikini-Todd, age 61**

Since receiving the laser treatment, I have noticed that I have been walking easier. The pain has diminished considerably and I do not wake up in the middle of the night with severe leg pains. I do not take a lot of time waking up and trying to rock myself out of bed every day. Putting on my shoes ceased to be an agonizing ritual. I don't groan when I drop something on the floor knowing picking it up will not be an epic undertaking. When I do my leg lifts, I don't creak like the Tin Man. Entering and emerging from the car does not require an imaginary forklift. Running after the grandkids is actually doable; cartoonish, but doable. It hasn't helped my dancing techniques but lasers can only do so much. Thank you, Dr. Alosa; your staff has been attentive, professional, and fun.
—**Dale La Forest, age 63**

I went for treatment with crutch and cane for three weeks. I finished my sixteenth day without the crutch and cane. I was in so much pain in my back, right hip down to my thigh, and numbness in my leg. After several laser treatments, the pain is less and no numbness. I'm glad I saw Dr. Jeremy Alosa's ad for pain relief from the class-4, deep-tissue laser. Thank you, Dr. Alosa, and your staff. I am able to sleep through the night, do

house chores, and go out with my friends. The laser treatment has helped me to do a lot of things.
—**Dolores Corpus, age 78**

I have a herniated disc in my lower right back. For years off and on I have had pain on the right side of my body. Just recently I could not get out of bed without getting pain on my right side. Getting up and down was very difficult because of the pain. At times I couldn't drive, exercise by walking, swimming, boogie boarding, or surfing. My right side was very tight and the muscles were tense and tight. Laser treatments helped the injury so I am able to be without pain.
—**Fred Quizon, age 68**

My lumbar spinal stenosis caused prickly numbness, cramping, and burning pain along the entire outer side of my left leg and foot. The numbness was ever present, the cramps intense at times, but it was the burning pain that led me to see Dr. Alosa. The treatments soothed the inflammation in my spine and gave me sweet relief from the burning pain. The numbness is not as severe and seems to have migrated to my calf and foot. The cramps are treatable with stretching exercises and extra hydration. I feel more confident and comfortable in my walking and maintaining my balance. I have more energy and can walk further and stay on my feet longer. Most of all, the laser therapy has relieved my burning pain which sopped my energy and depressed me. The treatments helped to brighten and improve my outlook on life.
—**Ellen Lim, age 79**

I am amazed! After just the first laser treatment on my lower back, I bent over to touch the ground—PAIN-FREE! After four auto accidents and incidental bodily pains in my back, legs, shoulder, and hands, and further treated with PE and acupuncture and additionally, had two knee replacements and two rotator cuff surgeries, I am very happy to be able to walk in comfort, PAIN-FREE, including able to do again veggie/flower/housework tasks. It's wonderful to be 85–90 percent pain-free and live comfortably every day now, driving pain-free when reversing, turning left, right, and parking; it's a pleasure to be nearly normal. Yard work is no longer a chore—to sit and move with ease and no longer need help to rise up. Dr. Alosa, please continue your wonderful laser treatment so others may recover enough to enjoy daily living again.

—Dorothy H. Yoshikawa, age 86

I have been suffering with pain in both of my kneecaps. I used to have my husband rub my knees so the pain will go away but the pain was still there. I was introduced to the laser treatment, deep tissue. I have been treated twice a week for my pain. I noticed my pain got less and less. Today, both knees are pain-free. Thank you, Dr. Alosa, and staff.

—Emma Ernestburg, Laie, HI, age 75

For many years my knees were painful but apparently not severe enough for surgery. To relieve the pain, I used many types of medical plasters and ointments. The laser treatments resulted in no pain anymore in the knee and occasional pain in the other knee. I am thus able to walk more comfortably and apparently with a more normal posture.

—Florence Pang, age 82

I tried acupuncture because I had lower back pain, and pain in my right knee and also my right lower leg. The pain is was not gone so I called Dr. Alosa's office to make an appointment to try this LiteCure laser treatment. After 16 treatments twice a month, my lower back pain is 75 percent gone, and I feel less pain to my right knee and lower leg.

—Filemon Cortez, age 71

After about my third laser treatment, I noticed that my condition pertaining to the severe pain in my legs/feet had improved about 80 percent. Now I no longer need to take my pain pills for my legs/feet three times a day. I can go without taking any pain pills for 6–8 days. When I need to take any, once a day is sufficient. The pain in my legs/feet has subsided to the extent where I feel much better physically and emotionally. I also feel more relaxed.

—Hilda Fo, age 93

I have been suffering from pain in my wrists and finger joints for more than 10 years. In the past few years, numbness developed, and pains were progressively getting worse. As a result of laser therapy, the numbness is almost gone and wrist pains are significantly reduced. I live more normally. I can now do several pushups.

—Hisako Koga, age 69

I have had treatments for two months, and the pain in my knees is almost 100 percent gone. I was skeptical about this treatment, so I'm so happy to have finally found something that helped me. Thank you. After these treatments I can now walk with no pain. I can climb stairs and walk for longer periods of time. Before this, I was using a cane; now I don t need it. I would strongly recommend this treatment.

—Idamae Hamasaki, age 68

Having arthritis at age 88 is not a feeling that anyone can enjoy. I tried other treatments and medication, but still the pain was there. I saw an ad in the newspaper, called, and made an appointment. I came in to see Dr. Alosa with pain in both knees and right shoulder. We started off with my right shoulder, and the second treatment was on my knees. After the treatment, I felt less pain, and I look forward to the next treatments. After each treatment I felt less pain in both knees, Going through the LiteCure laser treatment therapy is a great experience for me to overcome my pain Even though I still walk with my cane, my knees are more stable with less pain. The pain within my shoulder also subsided. What a wonderful feeling. I haven't felt this way for a long time. LiteCure laser treatment is the best therapy I have ever given to myself. It's a miraculous treatment. My body deserves the best. Mahalo, Dr. Alosa!

—Inocencio Cabrera, age 91

I had pain in my right hip joint, especially when walking. It started about two years ago and was getting worse. An X-ray revealed moderate to severe arthritis. The laser therapy helped to eliminate most of the dull aching pain in the area. However, I continue to have pain and difficulty walking and climbing stairs when I put my whole weight on my right leg. The laser treat-

ments decreased pain to the level where I can get up faster from a sitting position, walk around my home without the tendency to drag my right leg, and do housework with more ease. I recently declined an invitation to visit Japan because I felt that I could not keep up with them. I am hoping that with the combination of improvement with laser treatment and doing strengthening exercises, I can go on future trips.
—**Jane Miyabe, age 82**

I was previously taking 650 mg of Tylenol for arthritis to alleviate the pain in my knee. The laser treatments improved my knee by 95 percent. I am no longer taking the extra-strength Tylenol for pain. Looking forward to enjoyable trips without stressing about my knee pain.
—**Jerry Okuda, age 74**

The laser treatments have taken away most of the pain in my right shoulder and left elbow area. Without the persistent pain, I'm able to play golf again and get back to working out in the gym. I have a more positive and happy attitude towards life knowing that I can once again do things I enjoy.
—**Joseph Goulart, age 47**

I had problems with my foot, my knee, and my back, which made everyday work and life painful and difficult. Now the old feeling is back and I can get around again like I used to without the hurt. My foot feels better, standing and walking. My knee feels so much better. After having surgery and physical therapy, there was still pain. Now the pain is gone! I can go walk, work, play—whatever. Thank you!
—**Kanchana Owens, age 59**

I saw your advertisement in the newspaper and because I have arthritis in my knee I got interested in it and called in. The first treatment I had helped me, so I decided to go through the treatments. I've just completed the regimen. I'm not fully recovered as I expected, but I can walk around without pain. Once in a while I feel a little uncomfortable, but it's much better than before. I'm thankful I went through this treatment as I can walk around without pain.

—Kay Higuchi, age 85

I injured my left arm/elbow three months ago. Medical advice was to rest it, ice treatments, or heat. The pain would wake me during sleep, which made a good night of sleep difficult. After my first treatment with Dr. Alosa I felt immediate relief. Seventy-five percent of the pain was gone. At present, I am 80 percent pain-free.

—Kelly Ann Souza, age 49

About 15 years ago I sustained a shoulder injury playing tennis. My doctor gave me two choices: surgery or physical therapy and exercise. I opted for the physical therapy and exercise. After many months of painful therapy and exercise, my shoulder was well enough for me to get into some weight training three times per week. Eventually it led me to golf and I have been playing for the past 10 years. I would have frequent pains on the injured shoulder but mostly in the neck area. These would turn out to be painful neck aches. I continued to exercise and play golf through the discomfort. A few months ago I read an advertisement in the *Star Advertiser* about the LiteCure laser therapy and decided to try their trial visit. I was impressed that before the free treatment, Dr. Alosa (Alosa Family Chiropractic) asked me a series of questions and also checked my spine. I have been in twice a-week treatment for four weeks and the results have been quite amazing. I was relieved of some pain immediately. As of this writing I am now 80 percent pain-free in my neck area and have stopped taking pain medications. I also play golf pain-free and don't suffer the after-effects after a round. I am very happy with my decision to receive this laser therapy and would recommend this to anyone like me, suffering from past injuries.

—Ken Abe, age 68

My back was hurting until I read in the newspaper about laser treatment for the back by Dr. J. Alosa. After a few treatments my back felt better. By the fifteenth treatment the pains in my back had gone. I would like to thank Dr. Alosa and his assistant for the laser treatments they gave me.

—Larry Arakaki, age 88

My treatments started on April 15, 2011, with a treatment twice a week. After Dr. Alosa noticed improvement after a few weeks, he recommended once-a-week treatment. Since that time I have experienced more flexibility, less pain, and a better range of motion in my left knee. (I was diagnosed with osteoarthritis in my left knee in 2008.) I can honestly say it has given me more mobility in my knee and neck area. Now I'm able to stand for longer periods of time. The circulation and recovery time is less when I exert my muscles. Support and flexibility is what I really have been able to gain from treatments.

—Lawrence R. Ah-Nee Jr., age 60

After laser treatments I feel good and I'm more active again after years of pain in my lower back. Thank you, Dr. Alosa. I feel great; your laser treatments helped me tremendously. I'm 85 percent cured. I don't have pain in my lower back. I'm able to do more things at work and home. My quality of life has improved a lot. I highly recommend this treatment.

—Leo Ganal, age 73

Before I treated my knees with laser treatment, my knees were so bad and painful every time I walked. I believed that was the cause of my limping and slow walking. I took many different kinds of painkillers; aspirins never helped. So I decided to ask my doctor about the cortisone shot. I had that shot every four months and that really helped my pain. One day we saw an ad in the paper. It cost very little, so we decided to go and do it. It is so amazing after the first treatment. I know my knee pain is different. Both knees are getting better and better every day. Before I had this laser treatment, I hardly moved my knees. Now I go to the senior program every day and some days I help our supervisor instruct exercise to our elderly group. Wow! One day I jumped with two legs and I never felt any pain. AMAZING! And I believe they will get better after my full schedule of treatments. Mahalo and thank you to Dr. Alosa and all your staff! God bless!

—Lepeka Emosi, age 66

Please let me tell you how much your laser treatments have helped me. I am an 86-year-old woman who has suffered from lower back pain forever

and thought I would live in pain the rest of my life. After a free exam and treatment, and laser treatments, my pain is 95 percent gone. I would recommend anyone with any pain to go to see Dr. Jeremy Alosa first—not as a last resort. By doing laser treatment first, you feel better faster. Your treatment will be a treat. If Dr. Alosa's offices were a restaurant, he would get five stars. I now sit, knit, walk, dance as I did 60 years ago.
—Lillian Marks, age 88

The sharp pain under my patella has just about gone away and the pain/ache around the knees has greatly diminished. My backache and sciatica have also decreased a lot. I was having to take Aleve every day to be able to walk and work without limping noticeably. Now I can go without pills unless I do a lot of walking or carrying things. I can walk without pain perhaps 90 percent of the time.
—Lorna Park, age 64

From getting out of the bed in the morning and moving about, I always experienced pain in my lower back. It would go away as the day went by until I went to bed at night. Then it would be another cycle the next day, and so on. When Dr. Alosa started my laser therapy, it gradually eased my pain. Now I feel the strength and flexibility in my movements after several treatments. Thank you and I'm grateful for being pain-free, Dr. Alosa. I can get up in the morning feeling good; my walking distance has improved. I have more energy.
—Maria Straatman, age 64

Since receiving the deep-tissue laser treatments, my knee has improved significantly. In my opinion, I have about an 80 percent improvement, which is better than if I hadn't received this treatment. Walking up and down steps have been much easier. Even getting up from a sitting position improved tremendously. I believed.
—Marianne Omoto, age 80

I injured my left wrist in January 2011 and had to stop my golfing. Medical treatments were three cortizone shots and physical therapy with heat and ice treatments. I was also told to rest the wrist completely, wearing a brace almost 24 hours. The pain level was at a 9/10. After the first treatment with Dr. Alosa in June, 80 percent of the pain was gone. Completing my treatments, I am back to golf and 95 percent pain-free. I missed my golf activity very much and gardening. I can now do these activities without wearing a wrist brace.

—Marilyn Kosora, age 72

The two areas of treatment (left wrist and right heel) are almost completely pain-free. I started laser treatments only a month ago and am amazed that the pain is almost completely gone and that I am now able to put pressure on my heel and weight on my wrist. I've had these pains for nearly two years and went to a sports doctor who diagnosed me with tendon problems in my wrist and heel that also created a bone spur, and he referred me to a rehab center for treatments. However, the pain did not go away; but, instead, I was living with the pain until I decided to try laser treatments. I am amazed at the quick healing process and results. I informed my family and friends about this new technology in Hawaii that works so that they can also benefit from their ailments with pain. My body is no longer in consistent and persistent pain after the laser treatments. I feel better both physically and emotionally. I plan to start exercising again and doing the things I used to do and wasn't able to do for almost two years.

—Marvi Shibuya, age 58

The benefits I have received from the laser treatments prevented me from having my left knee surgery done. After the beginning of the laser treatment, I was able to stand up from the bed without pain. I was able to sleep on my side. Climbing up the stairs was much easier, without pain. The laser treatments made me want to help others, tell them of my laser treatment. The benefits improved my life with no knee surgery. Weeks of laser treatments have improved my life.

—May Castro, age 74

I have been having neck and shoulder pains for over 10 years. Gradually my right hands and fingers started to hurt and become numb. After several treatments, it seems 90 percent better. My numbness has gone away and I can move my neck with less pain. I'm also having leg problems, with pain, which keeps me awake at nights. Laser treatments have helped me a lot. I can do my daily things with less pain.

—May Shintani, age 79

For many years my arthritic left knee was painful. It was hard to walk very far without limping or having to sit down to ease the pain. With the laser treatments, I have been able to more without a dull ache, or once in a while, a sharp pain. I am able to get up with relative ease of motion. Best of all I am able to play tennis and coach without having to use a brace. I sleep better without getting up because of pain in my knee. I can walk up and down steps with relative ease. I am able to exercise by walking without pain, which also keeps my weight down. In general, because of the laser treatments, I am able to move about, walk better, and play sports.

—May Ann Beamer, age 73

I've been living with stiffness and limited mobility in my neck for the last three years. When I saw the advertisement in the *Star-Advertiser* about LiteCure class-4, deep-tissue laser treatment, I decided to give it a try. After the laser treatment, my neck is much more mobile and not as stiff Now I can turn my neck any which way much easier than before without as much pain and effort.

—Myles Takata, age 69

Laser therapy diminished my shoulder and rotator cuff pain by 75 percent. I could have done this treatment earlier if I had learned about it. It could have saved me money and eased my pain in such a shorter time. It has gotten me back to regular movements of the hand, specifically my finger flexibility and a little of my shoulder movements. With the soreness and pain diminished, I was able to do my regular activities. Although, for now, after the twelfth treatment, I still strive to lift my arm; it still hurts a bit.

—Norie Anne Nolasco, age 52

It made my finger joints on both hands, which had been stiff and sometimes locked up, to be okay now. Movement is normal and joints are not stiff. It improved greatly the right hand thumb's base joint; the thumb is still a bit stiff and moving the thumb is still painful. I learned much, such as dietary omega-3 oils help, and ice helps when my wrist is stiff and sore. Also, gentle stretching helps. I learned a wrist brace helps too, when I have to do lifting. I need my hands to work well, as my profession is cleaning. I don't want to have to find other work, as I love the job I have now and it supports me well. I don't want to have to turn to currently used arthritis medicine, which has side effects, is expensive, and doesn't cure the problem.

—Patricia Ayers, age 76

The arthritis pain in my left thumb and right shoulder was unbearable at times and I could not find any relief. I was skeptical about the laser treatment at first, but after the first treatment I realized that my pain in my shoulder was almost gone. After a few more treatments, my thumb joint was much better and I got almost all of the strength back, which I never thought would happen. It really works because it helps open the blood vessels and helps the body heal itself. I have the strength back in my hand again. I am not in constant pain and in need of drugs to relieve pain.

—Paul Lucas, age 66

Before treatments, I was limited in walking far and standing long hours. I was suffering from lower back pain and both knees hurt all the time, the right knee, more so. Before treatments, I was pretty much confined to the house; before that I was pretty active. I have done therapy at Castle Medical Center and have also done water therapy. All did nothing for me but take up my time. One day I was reading the newspaper and saw Dr. Alosa's ad. I said, "Why not?" and it was the best investment I made by far. I have been repeatedly seeing my regular MD for almost a year with constant pain every day in my lower back and both knees. Before doing the deep laser treatments, my doctor wanted me to do a full body bone scan at Queens Hospital to rule out everything including cancer, so I went and had it done. Queens did the wrong test on me and wanted me to go back. I did not want to do it again because of the nuclear medicine they put in you. I kept on with my deep laser treatments, went back to see my doctor, and my body did not show high infection in my body anymore. She asked me what was I doing, I know it was only the laser treatment so I told her. She said I did not have to take the bone scan again and she was not going to interfere with what was helping me. The laser treatments are awesome. I would highly recommend it to anyone who has pain.

—Paulette Soon, age 65

I feel just fine now, more than I ever was. Before, I spent a lot on other treatment, chiropractic, acupuncture, massage, neck stretching—it did not do any good. It only lasted for a while. Then I would just have to start all over again. I can walk longer without back or neck pain. The results of this treatment improved my life style in whatever I do. I feel energetic; I sleep well, walk well, work well on my family farm in Kahana Valley, using a shovel, pick, hoe, weed whacker, chair, saw, push wheelbarrow, without back or neck pain. I am glad that I took this treatment. I recommend that all who take this treatment take the full treatment.

—Peter Kau Kawaa Jr., age 73

I have less back and leg pain, more feeling of energy to go out and do things. I don't stoop over as much and I am sitting and standing straighter. I sleep better and don't mind exercising. I can now actually go out at night and dance longer and often. I look forward going to the YMCA to work out and stretch. Mostly the treatments have allowed me to live a more social life with my friends and family.

—Randall Lee, age 58

My wrist hurt when I brushed my teeth. I had to use both hands to turn the door knobs. I couldn't use the can opener and other things when I had to turn my wrist. Also, both thumb joints were painful along with my trigger fingers. I couldn't grasp anything without hurting. After the laser treatments I am able to do most of those things without asking for help. Now I can return to my exercise classes. I couldn't go down on the floor and stand up without the support of my hands. The strain was on my wrist. Dr.Alosa is a very caring person and so is his staff. Thank you, doctor.

—Rose Ching, age 90

I have had ankylosing spondilitis for the past 27 years. All these years, I have used all kinds of NSAID medications. Since I started my laser treatment, I stopped using Celebrex, thereby saving my kidney and liver. I can walk up the steps without using the handrails. My pain (ankles) literally went from 100 percent to 5 percent, which makes my husband less stressed. These benefits have given me a new lease on life. I used to wish to just be dead to escape from my pain. I asked God for a miracle and he gave me one. Thank you, Dr. Alosa. I wish I had found you a long time ago.

—Rowena Pilapil-Murphy, age 58

My left knee pain began in June 2010 while golfing at a local golf course. The low-grade pain and discomfort caused me to walk with a limp. After about four months of pain, I decided to try the LiteCure laser treatment. The pain and discomfort was reduced around 90 percent. Now, I walk without a limp and can walk 18 holes of golf without the pain and discomfort I used to have. However, there is a knocking sound of bone to bone sometimes, but there's no pain. Also, going up and down stairs is much easier.

—Roy Akaki, age 82

I am thankful for the laser treatments that took the pain away from my body. It took 20 treatments, but it was worthwhile. The treatments made me walk without pain. I am pain-free on my arm. I'm able to get out of bed without pain. I am thankful for this treatment.

—Sadie Honda, age 81

For many years I was under a doctor's care relative to my back pain running down my legs. After my laser treatments I do not feel any pain in my back or down my legs. I do not need my cane anymore and can walk rather nicely.

—Shuji Akiyama, age 91

The pain in my left knee from knee replacement is now about 80 percent less than when I came for laser treatment. I can walk and bend my knee much more than when I started. My right knee is about 85 percent less pain and is still very painful at times. I can now play golf much better and walk up hills and steps. I sleep at night much better also. I can bend my knee much more than before.

—Soo Lee, age 75

I got relief from being in pain almost/mostly every day. I would be taking Aleve about every other day just to be pain-free, so I could do my work as an auto mechanic. After getting the laser treatment for a couple months, I am about 80 percent free of pain, and I take Aleve maybe once every other week.

—Spencer Takaki, age 68

I am now 90 percent free from my lower back pain. I looked forward to each treatment because it resulted in a noticeable improvement to my lower back. Without the constant lower back pain, I now have a positive outlook. I can continue my daily activities and exercises and enjoy playing golf again.

—Stephen Watarai, age 68

I previously used a cane as a result of back surgery, but after the initial laser treatment, I no longer need to. My lower back pain and sciatica pain to my legs have been minimized. With each laser treatment, I continued to improve significantly. I am walking steadier and taller! I am able to do more in life than before receiving the laser treatments. I have a new lease on life! My family, friends and coworkers have noticed my transformation. Thank you very much, Dr. Alosa, and your staff, Casey and Jeannie. I'm 75 percent better, if not more. After 16 treatments, I have had about a 70 percent decrease in pain and greater range of motion in my feet and ankles. My posture has improved; I am walking better and with less pain, and I can wear shoes that did not fit for the past year. Thank you!

—Suzanne Enerson, age 72

I have been relieved of constant pain in my lower back, hips, buttocks, and legs. Tingling, and numbness on both feet is down to 1 percent. I can sleep well at night. I've been more cheerful and focused. The laser treatment has helped eliminate my pain 99 percent—most of the time. I thank Dr. Jeremy Alosa. Because of the laser treatment, my whole life has been free of pain. I have become more energetic and optimistic at 84 years old; I'm a senior citizen. Henceforth I plan to be active, but no strenuous vigorous activity. For all of this I am so grateful to Dr. Jeremy Alosa. The laser treatment does work. You, as the patient, must cooperate and take care of yourself.

—Teraza Fernandez, age 84

I received treatment for both knees due to an injury and arthritis. I was somewhat skeptical at the beginning but after the first treatment I immediately noticed a big difference in flexibility I didn't have before, so I became a believer because it worked. Before the laser treatment I could not sleep more than two hours at a time at night, the pain was so great. My knee felt at times like it was just dangling there; I could not bend it, or walk for any distance. After my treatments I have complete flexibility; I can walk without a noticeable limp and I can sleep thru the night now and get a good night's sleep. I would recommend the laser treatment to anyone suffering. It works.

—Ty Hooper, age 59

I have been suffering from back pain, mostly on the left side for a few years. After several laser treatments, my back increased muscle strength; it got better and better. Now after treatments, I felt 80 percent pain-free in my back. I do not have to take medication often. I can sit and stand longer and longer without pain. My sleeping is much better now. I can sleep freely on my back as long as I want. My numbness in the toes somehow does not bother me. I still get back pain sometimes, but I think that is related to my age. Thank you, Doctor Alosa and staff, who always treat patients nicely and respectfully.

—Van Trang Nguyen, age 62

I have had sciatic pain from my buttocks to my ankle since December 2010. Two and a half months of physical therapy helped to reduce 85 percent of the pain, but then improvement stopped. From the very first treatment, I could feel a sensation lessening the tightness in my calf area and ankle. The continued treatment has reduced pain to about 5 percent. I can now sleep through the night, and if I have to go to the bathroom I can return to bed and fall asleep without throbbing pain in my lower leg.
—**Warren Ah Loo, age 84**

I went to see Dr. Jeremy Alosa, DC on March 5th & 6th for the free trial and enjoyed the treatment. I was able to feel a little better and accepted the treatment. When we started the treatment on 3/12/13 & 3/14/13 the pain started to subside, but it would come back and I was limping. It was my right knee and the pain was still there. I would go home on the bus and sometimes I was in pain. As I continued treatment it started getting a little better. But I was in pain, but with treatments I was able to walk a little better and my limping started to get better. I'm able to walk and not need to replace my knee. I'm able to do my work around the house. I'm able to work on my house. I'm doing stretching exercises. I'm going on a trip with a lot of walking hopefully I will be able to enjoy myself to be pain free.
—**Caroline Ogawa, age 69**

When I first started treatments, I was suffering so much from neck pain, headaches and shoulder pain. After 5 weeks of treatment, headaches are 95% gone, neck pain is still there, and shoulder pain has gone down about 60%. When I get up in the morning, the pain is not as bad as it used to be. Now when I get up in the morning, I don' have headaches which kept me up at night. Neck pain is still there. My shoulder pain has gone down a lot. I can do more things now, such as doing my laundry. I can vacuum and do my gardening.
—**Lorraine Mosca, age 70**

Before laser treatments, my right hand, during the morning hours, I have pain, numbness, unable to make my hand into a fist because of swollen joints. After treatments, the pain has subsided. There is still a little pain and numbness. I am still unable to make a fist, but because there is less pain, I am able to get more sleep during the early morning hours. Less pain, since the laser treatments, allows me to be more functional with my right hand. It's an improvement from what it was before the treatments. Resulting in less pain and less stress.

—Harold Hong, age 79

I was always welcomed with a very pleasant smile and prompt treatment as scheduled with compassion and friendliness. Parking was always validated. The laser treatment was always warm, soothing, comfortable and relaxing. Thanks to the laser treatment, I'm able to sleep more comfortably without pain in my left and right shoulders as well as my thigh and leg. I spent the past weekend on the big island enduring the plane ride and long walks at the airport. A stressful weekend attending death in the family, I was able to cope without Advil or Tylenol. I came home with a knitting project that I would have never thought of getting started on. My treatment was longer than anticipated but, Dr. Jeremy Alosa, Emy and Liz did their very best to accommodate me with a very pleasant attitude. Mahalo Nui Loa for your warm and friendly help.

—Yoshi Kishinami, age 87

The most beneficial results I have received from the Deep Tissue Laser treatments is diminished pain in my knees and surrounding muscles and connecting tendons. My posture has improved. I walk with a steadier gait. The treatment enabled me to progressively perform more active water aerobic exercises & stretches. I can now drive without my right leg cramping. I am able to stay on my feet longer and walk a little farther without pain. One of the best results is that I am able to sleep through the night without pain waking me up in the wee hours. I feel better! I combined this treatment with weekly and then Bi-weekly Reflexology massage, which I feel has complimented the laser treatment. I have now resumed weekly Chair Yoga as part of my program.

—Barbara J Angelo, age 69

As a previous patient of Dr. Alosa for several years (he reversed a serious back condition) I was certain he could find a way to help with the worsening pain and swelling in my foot and heel. I also have osteoarthritis in my joints. I was very curious about this new laser therapy and so I signed up for a series of treatments. The first benefit I saw from the laser treatments was the reduction in swelling in my ankle and foot after about 4 sessions. Then the heel pain diminished greatly, and I could actually walk without a limp for the first time in several months. As the treatments progressed the pain and swelling was much less frequent so we moved the treatments to my joints. The discomfort was lessened and walking was much easier. I can now walk without a limp, and even after a long day at work, I am still not limping. There is significantly less swelling and inflammation. I can walk and stand longer than in previous months.

—Joyce Garnes, age 66

I had two back surgeries years ago, but still had to take Advil 3-4 times a day to alleviate the pain. I didn't want more surgeries so I decided to try the laser treatments. After a few sessions, I began to notice less pain. I started walking more erect without having to brace myself. Now I get up in the morning with a positive attitude. I can walk from room to room without holding on to the furniture and walls. I spend more time tending to my fish ponds, orchids and plants with much less pain.

—Alexander Fraser, age 72

I, Ruth, when I came to Dr. Alosa for treatment, I was 81 years old. I was an unhappy person that I wanted to go with my deceased husband. After receiving my laser treatment, I'm a happy person today. Thank you Dr. Alosa for the laser treatment. Now I'm 82 years old and pain free for my pinch nerve and arthritis. Thank you Dr. Alosa for the free extra treatments, you really made sure I'm pain free. If you are in pain go see Dr. Alosa or call Emy phone (808) 596-4800 for an appointment. Emy is very helpful, nice and friendly, so is Liz. Once again, thank you Dr. Alosa for the laser treatment. God Bless you and the staff.

—Ruth Shiratori, age 82

After completing your laser treatment program, the suffering of both hands of pain, numbness and tingling have reduced to a level that has made me feel a lot better. I have less pain as never before. Although I still have the numbness and tingling, I am functioning better than before the treatments. This treatment has made me feel better and I'm glad that I took it. I may not be a 100%, but I am able to sleep longer without having to wake up several times a night from pain in my hands. It doesn't take me as long to button my shirt anymore. I am now able to apply pressure to my fingertips without much pain.
—Mariano Rellin, age 80

In my old age, I have to contend with a number of chronic health problems, particularly ambulatory, i.e. falling. One of the contributing factors is arthritis in my lower back. Laser treatments have minimized the pain. I am now able to continue exercise activities at the YMCA with the assistance of the trainer who is helping with strengthening my legs.
—George Nishimura, age 84

My right knee would have pain and stiffness going down stairs, getting out of bed in morning, driving for long periods or just sitting. With treatment to my right knee, I can now walk down stairs – wake up in morning and get out of bed with no problem – also I can sit and drive for long periods and stand up and walk with no problem, a 100% difference. Left thumb joint was stiff, weak and at times in pain – with treatments – no stiffness and pain. Laser treatments on my right knee have me walking down stairs, climbing up ladders with no pain or stiffness. On my left thumb it has stopped the stiffness and pain I had and be able to work with tools better without stiffness and more flexibility.
—Randy Wong, age 60

I suffered for several years with increasing arthritis pain in my hands, neck, back, and knees. Numerous visits to the doctors, acupuncturists, and chiropractors resulted in only temporary relief. I went to see Dr. Alosa regarding his advertisement in the Star Advertiser. After the interview and first treatment I decided to take the full treatment. After the treatments by Dr. Alosa's trained staff, I noticed a reduction in my pains. The Class IV Deep Tissue Laser treatments have reduced them by 60% - 75%. I have enjoyed meeting with his staff and their compassion and friendliness towards me. Also, most importantly is the promptness in their scheduled appointments.

—Marlene

I had pain in both knees when walking up and down my drive way. Since going to laser treatments, pain has subsided by 50% - 75%. Walking is much more comfortable now. Being able to go up and down my drive way to pick up my mail and take out the trash bin with ease is a blessing.

—Kirby Loo, age 89

Before I started the laser treatment, I could barely move my fingers because they were so painful. Now with the treatment the pain is at a minimum or non-existent. I can now hold objects in my hands, as before it was so bad that everything I had in my hands were falling down. I can make a fist with no pain.

—Elvia Aragon, age 66

I regained full function of my neck and lower back. I have noticed a big difference in my lower back. I used to have severe pain running down the back of my right leg down to my knee, making it very difficult for me to bend over to get out of bed. Now I am able to do all the things that I used to do without the unbearable pain running down the back of my right leg and knee. The pain in my neck would cause me to have a stiff neck and restrict me from being able to turn my head all the way. Now I am able to turn and tilt my head freely without the severe pain. The benefits from the laser treatments have helped me to move freely without any restrictions and pain. I am able to sit, stand and get out of bed without any problems due to my lower back. As for my neck, I am able to sleep and sit at my computer without being in pain or waking up with a stiff and sore neck at least two or more times in a month. Now I have not had any of those problems.

—Teri Muraoka, age 32

The benefits I received from the laser treatment regarding the arthritis in my right knee were very beneficial. I'm able to walk up the stairs without feeling much pain like before. I also noticed that my ankles are not as swollen. It's something about the laser treatment that brought down the swelling in both ankles. I am also getting out of bed easily without feeling any pain in my right knee. Also, I can no longer hear a clicking sound in my right knee. These benefits improved my life the most by bringing down the swelling in my ankles as well as relieving the pain in my right knee. This is something that I have struggled with for many years. I am also able to walk for a longer period of time, and climb many stairs in my home without any difficulty. Thank you Dr. Alosa and staff for being there for my daughter Teri as well as myself. I will proudly recommend your Light Cure Laser Therapy to my family and friends because you have saved me from having surgery on my right knee.
—**Sandra Muraoka, age 66**

After treatments I am able to do many things that I haven't been able to do before. These are to include: relief of pain, work in yard/garden, able to get up easier from a sitting position, get out of bed in the morning, and tie my shoes. It makes my day easier and I am able to do lots more than before. I can now play with my grandchildren.
—**James Mosca, age 70**

Arthritis had caused my right hand, wrist and fingers to be very stiff and painful. I decided to try the Deep Tissue Laser treatments that Dr. Alosa advertised. I noticed some improvement right away, and now that I have completed treatments, I can use my hands to do minor tasks without any pain. My hands and fingers movement have improved 85%. The treatments are painless and the doctor's office is staffed with very friendly and qualified people! I highly recommend the Deep Tissue Laser treatments!
—**Carolyn Kemble, age 94**

When I accompanied my husband for his first treatment for his arthritic shoulder, I had no intentions of being treated. During his interview I was curious if the laser treatment would relieve the pain in my Achilles tendon which I strained while bowling. At first, I was unsettling to go through the full treatment because I had my doubts. After 8 sessions my Achilles felt better but I still experienced some pain so I elected to continue through eight more sessions. My Achilles is not 100 percent pain free but it is better. At least I can continue the active lifestyle that I am used to.

—Carmen Padilla, age 70

After a few treatments my back pain was noticeably less, after 16 treatments I needed only half as much NSAIDS (Ibuprofen and Acetaminophen) as before to control my back pain. This effect has continued for almost three months from my last treatment, however I have recently noticed more back pain again and I'm not sure of the cause and effect. This laser treatment showed me that something noninvasive could be done to help and now I am beginning to pursue getting in better shape i.e. going to the gym, hiking again and no longer just freezing up and giving up because of my arthritis pain. I am beginning to believe these are things I can do to get back in shape and be able to function fully again without debilitating pain.

—Donovan Duncan, age 66

Having a positive attitude, I was able to gain a lot of satisfaction from my laser treatments. The pain decreased the more treatments I received. I could stand up without reaching for the walls, my cane or my walker all the time. I can now walk further and for longer periods of time which I finally felt the laser heal. I felt more at ease and less pressure around my knee joints. I am able to exercise for several minutes with leg lifts and knee bends. I walk from 10-15 minutes at a time. I enjoy my swimming, walking and aerobic classes twice weekly. I have managed to lose weight and maintain it so there is a lot less pressure on my knees. I can bend and scoot down too. I feel that the laser treatments have improved my pain, which is now 60% better most of the time.

—Rawlette P. Kraut, age 64

The deep tissue laser treatment improved my sore neck and shoulders. There is still some soreness when tuning my neck left and right. The amount of neck turning though did improve. My assessment on my

condition is about 50% improvement from the treatment. The treatment enables me to continue my favorite sport of golfing.
—**Arthur Shak, age 79**

I have less pain and can walk 70% better. I can walk much better and much further than when I started. I have a lot less pain in my right knee.
—**Donald Rudd, age 82**

After seeing my doctor he told me that I had arthritis in both of my knees, so he gave me Osteo Bi-Flex and Flexitol. Take and did not help at all. I met with Dr. Alosa and his laser treatment and now I have less pain in both knees. Laser treatment has lead me to be able to walk better, do the yard work and take my car out instead of just watching TV!
—**Moses Aweau, age 83**

Before seeing Dr. Alosa for laser treatment, I was in much pain in my artificial hip replacement 40 years ago; which came out of the socket causing pain. After receiving the full treatment I am 80% better – pain is still there but not as intense. I am able to sit and move with less pain. I can walk sometimes without the pain, at least now I am able to sit with less pain, too.
—**Dorothy Quizon, age 91**

Prior to receiving laser treatments, I need to take pain killers twice a day to relieve the pain in my hips and recurring down my right leg. Since undergoing this treatment I believe my pain has subsided by at least 75% and I am able to walk with the assistance of a walker.
—**Laura Loo, age 85**

I have arthritis in my right knee and had difficulty in walking up and down the stairs. After receiving the laser treatments I now am able to do the stairs without much difficulty including just walking for exercise. I play golf and the benefit I received is that I previously had a problem walking up and down hilly area without pain. In fact, I had to walk sideways like a crab. Now, after the laser treatments I can walk up and down the hill like a normal person and enjoy playing golf although my scores are bad.

—Terrance Lee, age 72

I have been suffering severe back pain for the past 3 years. I couldn't sit for a long time, bend over or reach for things without having sharp pain and numbness in my back and legs. I would limp when I walked and sometimes would have to crawl because the pain would be so bad. I came and saw Dr. Alosa for laser treatment to see if he could help me. Now I have no more pain. Laser treatments have brought me back to a younger age. I am now able to carry heavy things, do more activities than before, bend and reach for things with no more pain, and I do not limp any more. Now my wife doesn't have to hear me complain.

—Samuel B. Cadiz, age 70

References

Alexandratou, E., Yova, D., Handris, P., Kletsas, D. and Loukas, S. "Human Fibroblast Alterations Induced by Low Power Laser Irradiation at the single cell level Using Confocal Microscopy." Photochemical. *Photobiology.* Sci. 1, 2002, 547-552.

Anders, J.J., Geuna, S. and Rochkind, S. "Phototherapy Promotes Regeneration and Functional Recovery of Injured Peripheral Nerve." *Neurology.* Res. 2004 26, 233-239.

Angell, Marcia. *The Truth About the Drug Companies.* New York: Random House, 2004.

Babcock, D.F., Herrington, J., Goodwin, P.C., Park, Y.B. and Hill, B. "Mitochondrial Participation in the Intracellular Ca++ Network. J." *Cell Biology 1997, 136,* 833-844.

Bjordal JM, and Couppe C. "What is Optimal Dose, Power Density and Timing for Low Level Laser Therapy In Tendon Injuries?" A Review of in Vitro and in Vivo Trials. Department of Physiotherapy Science, University of Bergen, Norway. Abstract from the 7th International Congress of European Medical Laser Association, Dubrovnik, Croatia, June 2000.

Bjordal JM, Johnson MI, Lopes-Martins RA, Bogen B, Chow R, and Ljunggren AE. 2007. "Short term Efficacy of Physical Interventions in Osteoarthritic knee pain: A systematic review and Meta-analysis of Randomized Placebo-Controlled Trials." *BMC Musculoskeletal Discord 8;*51.

Burroughs, Stanley. *The Master Cleanse.* New York: Bourroughs Books. 1993.

Byrnes, K.R., Barna, L., Chenault, V.M., Waynant, R.W., Ilev, I. K., Longo, L., Miracco, C., Johnson, B. and Anders, J.J. 2004. "Photobiomodulation Improves Cutaneous Wound Healing in an Animal Model of Type II Diabetes." *Photomed. Laser Surgery. 22,* 281-290.

Campana V, Satsel A, Vidal AE, et al. 1993. "Prostaglandin E2 in Experimental Arthritis of Rats Irradiated with HeNe laser." *J Clin Laser in Med & Surg; 11:*79-81.

Campbell, Colin, Campbell, Thomas II. *The China Study.* Dallas, TX. Benbella Books, 2006.

Capaldi, R.A. 1990. "Structure and Function of Cytochrome C Oxidase." Annu. Rev. *Biochem. 59,* 569-596.

Chow, R.T. and Barnsley, L. "2005 Systematic Review of the Literature of Low Level Laser Therapy in the Management of Neck Pain." *Lasers Surg. Med. 37,* 46-52.

Cohen, Jay. *Overdose The Case Against the Drug Companies.* New York: Putnam Books, 2001.

Curtis, Clare, et. al., "Pathologic Indicators of Degradation and Inflammation in Human Osteoarthritic Cartilage are Abrogated by Exposure to N-3 Fatty Acids." *Arthritis & Rheumatism. Vol. 46,* Issue 6, 2002, 1544-1553.

De Castro E Silva Jr. O, et al. "Laser Enhancement in Hepatic Regeneration for Partially Hepatectomized Rats." *Lasers in Surgery and Medicine. 2001. 29* (1):73-77

Eddy, David. "Where is the Wisdom?" *British Medical Journal, 1991, 303*:798.

"Eighteen year follow up in the Veterans Affairs Cooperative Study of Coronary Artery Bypass Surgery for stable angina. The VA Coronary Bypass Surgery Cooperative Study Group." *Circulation 86* (1992): 121-30

"Eleven Year survival in the Veterans Administration randomized trial of coronary bypass surgery for stable angina. The Veterans Administration Coronary Artery Bypass Surgery Cooperative Study Group." *New England Journal of Medicine 311* (1984): 1333-339

Enwemeka CS and Reddy GK. "The Biological Effects of Laser Therapy and other Modalities on Connective Tissue Repair Processes." *The Journal of Laser Therapy, Vol. 12.* World Association of Laser Therapy. 2000.

Gigo-Benato, D., Geuna, S. and Rochkind, S. 2005 "Phototherapy for Enhancing Peripheral Nerve Repair. A review of the literature." *Muscle Nerve 31,* 694-701.

Goldberg, Robert, Katz, Joel. "A Meta-analysis of the Analgesic Effects of Omega-3 Polyunsaturated Fatty Acid Supplementation for Inflammatory Joint Pain." *Pain.* May 2007, *129* (1-2), 210-223.

Grossweiner, L.I. 2005 *The Science of Phototherapy: An Introduction.* Heidelberg: Springer Verlag.

Haley, Daniel. *Politics in Healing.* Washington, DC: Potomac Valley Press, 2000.

Hawthorne, Fran. *Inside the FDA*. Hoboken: John Wiley & Sons, 2005.

Honmura A, Ishii A, Yanase M, et al. 1993. "Therapeutic Effect of GaAIAs Diode Laser on Experimentally Induced Inflammation in Rats." *Lasers in Surg & Med: 13:* 463-469

Hopkins JT, McLoda TA, Seegmiller JG, and David Baxter G. 2004. "Low-Level Laser Therapy Facilitates Superficial Wound Healing in Humans: A Triple Blind, Sham-Controlled Study." *J Athl Train 39:* 223-229

Kassirer, Jerome. *On the Take*. New York: Oxford Press, 2005.

Lubart R, Friedman H, and Lavie R. "Photobiostimulation as a Function of Different Wavelengths. "*The Journal of Laser Therapy. Vol 12*. World Association of Laser Therapy. 2000.

Montesinos, M., et al. 1988. "Experimental Effects of Low Power Laser in Encephalin and Endorphin Synthesis. Laser." *Journal Eur. Med Laser Assn.; 1* (3): 2-7.

Moseley, Bruce, et. al., "A Contolled Trial of Arthroscopic Surgery for Osteoarthritis of the Knee." *N Engl J Med, Vol 347,* No.2, July 11, 2002.

Moynihan, Ray. Cassels, Alan. *Selling Sickness*. New York: Avalon, 2005.

Mrowiec, J., et al. 1997. "Analgesic Effect of Low Power Infrared laser Radiation in Rats." *Proc SPIE. Vol 3198:* 83-89.

Nickelston, Perry, "The Light Answer." *Advance for Physical Therapy & Rehab Medicine,* December 28, 2009.

Nicolau, RA., Martinez, M.S., Rigau, J. and Tomas, J. 2004. "Neurotransmitter Release Changes Induced by Low Power 830 nm Diode Laser Irradiation on the Neuromuscular Junctions of the Mouse." *Lasers Surg. Med. 35,* 236-241.

Ozner, Michael. *The Great American Heart Hoax*. Dallas, TX. Benbella Books, 2008.

Pryor, Brian. "Advances in Laser Therapy for the Treatment of Work Related Injuries." *Current Perspectives in Clinical Treatment & Management in Workers Compensation Cases,* 2011, 191-201.

Riegel, R., & Prior, B. 2008. "Clinical Overview and Applications of Class IV Therapy Lasers."

Sears, Barry. *The Omega Zone*. Regan Books, 2002.

Starfield, Barbara. "Is U.S. Health Really Best in the World?" *JAMA,* July 26, 2000, vol. 284, No. 4.

Stoll, Andrew, *Omega-3 Connection.* Simon & Schester, 2001.

Theodosakis, Jason. *The Arthritis Cure.* New York: St. Martins Griffin, 1997.

Trowbridge, John. *The Yeast Syndrome.* New York: Bantam Books, 1986.

Tuner, Jan. Hode, Lars. *Laser Therapy.* Grangesberg, Sweden: Prima-books, 2002.

Vickers, J., & Harrington, P. 2009. "Class IV Lasers: Maximizing the Primary Effects of Laser Therapy."

2 FREE
LASER TREATMENTS

CALL
(808) 596-4800

(For first time patients only)

Offer includes:

Diagnostic Exam, 2 Laser Treatments,
X-rays (If needed)

Printed in the USA
CPSIA information can be obtained
at www.ICGtesting.com
JSHW012032140824
68134JS00033B/3014

9 781599 324234